Psyched

Psyched

Seven Cutting-Edge Psychedelics Changing the World

AMANDA SIEBERT

foreword by
Julie Holland, MD

GREYSTONE BOOKS
Vancouver/Berkeley/London

Greystone Books Ltd.
greystonebooks.com

Cataloguing data available from Library and Archives Canada
ISBN 978-1-77164-879-0 (pbk.)
ISBN 978-1-77164-880-6 (epub)

Editing by Jennifer Croll
Copy editing by Brian Lynch
Proofreading by Dawn Loewen
Cover and text design by Belle Wuthrich

Printed and bound in Canada on FSC® certified paper at Friesens.
The FSC® label means that materials used for the product have been
responsibly sourced.

Greystone Books thanks the Canada Council for the Arts, the British
Columbia Arts Council, the Province of British Columbia through the
Book Publishing Tax Credit, and the Government of Canada for
supporting our publishing activities.

Canada

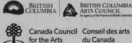
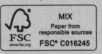

Greystone Books gratefully acknowledges the xʷməθkʷəy̓əm (Musqueam),
Sḵwx̱wú7mesh (Squamish), and səl̓ílwətaʔɬ (Tsleil-Waututh) peoples on
whose land our Vancouver head office is located.

Let this book be an expression of my gratitude
to every steward, keeper, and teacher; to every plant,
entheogen, and derivative; to Mother Earth for giving us
exactly what we need; and to every reader with a willingness
to examine that which exists beyond the mind.

May all of this be for the highest good.

———————

DISCLAIMER

———————

THIS BOOK IS not intended to be a substitute for medical advice from physicians. The reader should regularly consult a physician about matters relating to their health, and particularly with respect to any symptoms that may require diagnosis or medical attention. While this book may mention specific psychedelic drugs and associated compounds, the author and publisher recommend that readers consult with a medical professional if they are thinking about consuming psychedelics for a health-related purpose.

Although the author and publisher have made every effort to ensure that the information in this book was correct at press time, they do not assume, and hereby disclaim, any liability to any part for any loss, damage, or disruption caused by errors or omissions, whether such errors or omissions result from negligence, accident, or any other cause. The state of psychedelic research is evolving daily, and with the renewed interest in these compounds, more rigorous study will only continue. As such, future research on the topics discussed may come to conclusions that are contrary to what has been printed in this book.

Contents

FOREWORD

"MAY YOU LIVE in interesting times," goes the blessing and the curse.

Recent years have been both interesting and stressful for humanity. At times, our future has seemed uncertain. We have seen pandemics, wars, and an enormous shift from lives lived in the real world to lives lived online. And because we have become the worldwide-wired, we are now capable of witnessing ever more trauma. Marshall McLuhan warned us that with new technologies, our nervous system would no longer stop at the outline of our bodies. And so we're left with a reality where we're nearly always online, plugged into the world's trauma—and, perhaps not surprisingly, experiencing record levels of psychiatric symptoms. In 2019, U.S. depression and anxiety rates were 6.5 percent and 8 percent, respectively. In 2022, the Centers for Disease Control reported increases to 23 percent and 28 percent.

But the present day also offers some innovative solutions to our problems: new psychedelic-assisted therapies. The *New York Times* has run several glowing articles about the promise of psychedelic-assisted psychotherapy, including its use in treating post-traumatic stress disorder, depression, and addictive processes. Even *Good Housekeeping* and *Town & Country* have joined in. As we hear about an alphabet soup of novel drugs, the financial sector is aflutter with the prospects. There are intellectual property fights a-brewin' in the Wild West of drug development as new pharmacological entities are introduced and older, classic psychedelics get a chemical tweaking.

It makes sense that we, as a culture, are increasingly open to "outside the box" trauma treatments. Many of us are in pain; some mourn for lost ways of life, and even for the demise of our planet. But there is hope, and it can be found in these pages. The seven substances that Amanda Siebert details in *Psyched* offer change we can believe in. These mind-manifesting, heart-opening medicines can help us to heal our bodies and our souls. They can help us to explore our past or envision our future, to prioritize relationships and love and compassion. And they can help us to feel more connected to nature, the earth, and the cosmos.

All of the plant medicines and fungi in this book, and the synthetic drugs as well, can help to shift the brain into a more open and plastic state. Neuroplasticity is the remodeling of the brain. It happens whenever we learn, grow, and change. Exercise and antidepressants can induce neuroplasticity, and so can psychedelics. In this state, not only can well-worn ruts melt away, to be replaced by new paths, but different parts of the brain can communicate when before they had not. Other parts—the self-absorbed ones that never seem to quiet down—finally go offline for a while. Importantly, perspectives shift, and things are seen anew with fresh eyes and an open mind.

The seven transformational medicines in *Psyched* populate my "interesting times" as a psychiatrist. Finally, we have some more effective "breakthrough therapies" (as MDMA and psilocybin were designated by the FDA) to offer people in real psychic pain. We have spiritual medicines to help us find our way back to ourselves, and anti-inflammatory medicines to treat neurodegenerative diseases. There is much to be discovered in this world of post-traumatic growth.

As with any treatment, we (both clients and practitioners) have a responsibility to educate ourselves about the risks and the benefits of psychedelics. And that is why Siebert's well-researched, measured explanation and advice in these pages are so important. Please don't just read *Psyched*: discuss it with the explorers in your life. Teach them about drug testing, about safer use. Just as Siebert does, please emphasize harm reduction and consent and especially integration, because it's what we do after the session that really matters. Trauma needs to be processed, worked through, and made part of a bigger whole. That cannot be rushed—but it can, and should, be shared.

Likewise, it takes time to build a psychedelic community, but as Siebert shows in *Psyched*, there is room for us all: seekers, healers, researchers, disruptors, educators, lovers. We are all on the same page, not only now, in the reading of this sentence, but in seeking transcendence as part of our spiritual journey.

—JULIE HOLLAND, MD

Introduction

HOW OUR ATTITUDE
TOWARD PSYCHEDELICS
HAS EVOLVED

*Psychedelics are illegal not because a loving government
is concerned that you may jump out of a third-story window.
Psychedelics are illegal because they dissolve opinion
structures and culturally laid down models of behavior
and information processing. They open you up to the
possibility that everything you know is wrong.*
—Terence McKenna

PSYCHEDELICS HAVE REEMERGED as one of the twenty-first
century's most powerful sources of human improvement and
healing. While the wave of support for these medicines is
growing in mainstream society, the use of psychedelics—particularly sacramental and medicinal plants and fungi—dates
to prehistory. Psychedelic drugs and plant medicines can offer
new perspectives on treating illness—ones that create lasting,
positive change in people's lives, sometimes removing the need
for other medications. But that's just the beginning.

As we acquaint (or reacquaint) ourselves with these largely
plant-based substances that have been used throughout human
existence to bring better health, a clearer mind, and a more

pleasurable existence, context is crucial. This book seeks to highlight how psychedelics can enhance our health and wellness, while bridging the perceived gaps between their historical, social, cultural, and medical uses, through a lens informed by research, expert commentary, real-life stories from people who use psychedelics, and nearly ten years of my own life-changing experience.

My Personal Connection to Psychedelics

I FIRST USED psychedelics a decade ago, with absolutely no intention of self-improvement and not a clue of how profoundly they were about to alter my life's course. Together with a small group of trusted friends, I ate 2.5 grams (give or take) of magic mushrooms. We listened to music, made pastel art, and walked to the ocean, where I swore that for the first time I could see the sparkling pulsation of life in each and every organism that found its home on the beach. I experienced a feeling of interconnectedness to everything I encountered that day, from my friends to the critters along the shore and the artists playing music through our speakers, and while I certainly ate those mushrooms in the spirit of "recreation," it brought a deep sense of meaning to my life, and one that would impact me from that point forward (though I didn't know it at the time). Since my initial experience, I've journeyed with psilocybin many more times, sometimes with a friend or two, sometimes in complete solitude in nature, and at other times seated in a circle during a group ceremony. No matter what circumstances I've found myself in while exploring hidden realms of my subconscious (whether the trip was "good" or "bad"), one thing has proven to be consistent: each experience creates an opportunity for me to assess my life from the inside out (or, say, from the perspective of my higher self) and make conscious decisions to improve it.

My early experiences with psychedelics were positive, but my interest in using psychedelics to heal began in 2017, when I was diagnosed with PTSD (post-traumatic stress disorder), depression, and anxiety after coming to terms with sexual trauma I experienced in my early twenties. Later that year, I experienced an earth-shattering breakup and was convinced that my life as I knew it was over. Between the violent flashbacks and gut-wrenching heartbreak, I regularly fantasized about ending my life. When my psychiatrist prescribed selective serotonin reuptake inhibitors, or SSRIs, I was hesitant. A few years earlier, I'd watched my mother struggle to find the right one and didn't want to endure the laundry list of side effects she had, especially for a medication that might not work for me. Instead, I took the prescription to my family doctor, along with a printed copy of a recent study conducted at Johns Hopkins University and a stack of introductory notes I'd made while reading about something called "microdosing" with psilocybin. Microdosing is the practice of consuming a psychedelic in such low doses that its hallucinogenic effects are not felt. In my research, I had read anecdotal reports from people who had traded their daily antidepressant regimen in for capsules of powdered magic mushrooms or vials of liquid LSD, and I wondered if I could avoid antidepressants altogether. Thankfully, my doctor was already aware of some of the trials being conducted on psilocybin and gave me the green light to experiment with microdosing, as long as I scheduled a return visit in a few weeks.

While there isn't concrete data on the efficacy of microdosing, I experienced an almost immediate silencing of the voice that was always telling me life would be better if I wasn't around. Once that voice became quiet, I was able to tune in to what it was that I really needed: a sense of unconditional love for myself. Over the years, several plant medicines have helped me cultivate that love, particularly ayahuasca and San Pedro (two plant medicines often described as "the grandmother" and "the grandfather"). It was in group settings surrounded by strangers who grew quickly into friends where I came face-to-face with myself and discovered that not only was life worth living—it was worth embracing.

In addition to my own experiences, and to the wide variety of groundbreaking research papers and trials I've written about as a journalist, the personal testimonies I've heard describing both tangible and lasting improvements in quality of life are not small in number. Having a profound psychedelic experience might seem clichéd, but these stories never get old, and no two are the same—even when the same person uses the same compound in the same setting. It takes guts to dive headfirst into a psychedelic experience, but it also takes preparation, a safe and supportive container or setting for that experience, and integration (a term used widely in psychedelic-assisted psychotherapy to describe the process of understanding a nonordinary state of consciousness and then applying the lessons learned to everyday life).

In the wrong setting, a psychedelic journey has the potential to create harm, and while steps can be taken to mitigate that harm, I'm not here to gloss over those risks. Psychedelics are *not* a panacea, and if you are thinking of using them, there are a considerable number of factors to weigh before making the jump. I'm saying this as an individual who has benefited *immensely* from using psychedelics, in ways I sometimes find hard to comprehend given the limited number of treatment options currently available to those of us struggling with mental health issues. In conjunction with therapy, a healthy diet, regular exercise, and a regimented schedule prioritizing rest and self-care, experiences with psychedelics like psilocybin and ayahuasca helped me overcome debilitating diagnoses (along with a debilitating sense of worthlessness). While I have experienced profound improvements to my quality of life and tapped into a beautiful community of people both at home and around the world, I recognize that they are powerful drugs that must be approached with reverence and caution. While the drugs help facilitate healing, it's all the other pieces of the puzzle that make the work stick: support, community, a balanced lifestyle, and ample time to integrate the lessons that come from these powerful plant (and fungus) teachers.

The Psychedelic Renaissance

OVER THE LAST DECADE, the public view of psychedelics has been refreshed as scientific research has surged and the substances have received attention from some of the world's most respected academic minds and institutions. Drugs like MDMA and psilocybin have been granted breakthrough therapy designations by the U.S. Food and Drug Administration (FDA), a designation that expedites the development of drugs that treat serious or life-threatening conditions. In addition, several major universities, such as New York University and the University of California, Los Angeles, have dedicated new programs to the study of psychedelics, while new academic centers focused on psychedelics have opened around the world, signaling a second wave.

While research gains momentum, grassroots initiatives have led to legislative changes: several American cities, such as Ann Arbor, Detroit, Oakland, Santa Cruz, Seattle, and Denver, have decriminalized plant medicines, while the state of Oregon has legalized the therapeutic use of psilocybin. In this more tolerant atmosphere, public companies specializing in psychedelics are popping up all over, each promising to use shareholder money to build clinics, fund research, and create intellectual property and novel compounds—drugs we've never heard of before—for an ever-expanding list of ailments.

Although they are still being rigorously studied, psychedelics are becoming widely accepted by academics, physicians, and entrepreneurs as having potential in treating mental health disorders such as depression, anxiety, PTSD, and substance use disorder. The results of recent studies suggest that psilocybin could help treat major depressive disorder, and that it reduces end-of-life anxiety in cancer patients. Another suggests that LSD could lead to the reduction and even cessation of alcohol consumption among patients with alcohol use disorder. In patients with severe depression, ketamine has been shown to help with suicidal ideation. One study conducted by the Multidisciplinary Association for Psychedelic Studies (MAPS) found that patients with PTSD who underwent several rounds of MDMA-assisted psychotherapy were more likely to recover than those in a placebo group. This is just a tiny sample of the academic research into psychedelic therapy. As I write these words, dozens of institutions and firms are working on proving psychedelic hypotheses of their own.

Given what we know now about psychedelics, you may ask yourself, "Why did it take us so long to get here?" The answer to this question cannot be summed up in a single sentence. Layers of nuance, years of stigma, and campaigns of misinformation contributed to why modern medicine had all but abandoned the study of psychedelics after the late 1960s. Now that we're letting go of our long-held biases, the importance of these compounds to society is being revealed.

Contributions
to Society

NO MATTER HOW you feel about them, psychedelic drugs have had a profound and immeasurable influence on the world. In the '60s, they influenced a generation of people to rise up against their governments to protest war and unjust laws, and to fight for peace and civil rights. Looking at the art, music, and lifestyle of people who lived during this era, it's plain how psychedelia spurred massive cultural change.

While psychedelics had a huge impact on artists and activists, their use also made waves among intellectuals and academics, from inventors and technologists to scientists and mathematicians. Without LSD, we might not have the personal computer or the iPhone.[1] Inventors like Steve Jobs and Bill Gates admitted to using the classic psychedelic to help inspire their technological creations. Francis Crick, the Nobel Prize–winning scientist who discovered the double-helix structure of DNA, and John C. Lilly, the neuroscientist who first mapped the pain and pleasure pathways in the brain, also admitted to using LSD during their research.[2, 3] Mathematicians from Pythagoras to Ralph Abraham used mind-expanding substances to help work through problems and generate new ideas.[4, 5]

Some even more "out-there" ideas about the influence of psychedelic drugs suggest that Moses was high on DMT, or N,N-dimethyltryptamine, contained in the bark and leaves of the acacia tree when he received guidance from God to write the Ten Commandments.[6] (Benny Shanon, an Israeli professor of cognitive psychology, published a paper on this theory in the journal *Time and Mind* in 2008, though it was not exactly well received by Orthodox rabbis.) Researchers Terence and Dennis McKenna's "stoned ape" theory suggests the consumption of psychedelic mushrooms contributed to the significant growth in brain size between early *Homo sapiens* and our predecessors, *Homo erectus.*[7]

For the vast number of diverse Indigenous cultures that revere psychedelic plants and/or fungi as medicines of the most high, with divine qualities—the Shipibo and ayahuasca, the Mazatec and mushrooms, the Native American Church and peyote, and many, many more—these are not compounds that can lead to greater physical, mental, and emotional wellness, but sacred teachers that bring messages from God. In these communities, relationships with the divine are shaped and formed through ritualistic use of psychedelic plant medicines.

From Early Study to Illegality

CONSIDERING THE CONTRIBUTIONS these powerful substances have made to society, along with their potential for improving mental health and wellness, it's curious to see what led to their prohibition in the first place. While it didn't all happen at once, a series of events in the '60s and early '70s ensured that psychedelics would be swept under the rug for decades.

While the first wave of psychedelic research didn't rise up until the 1950s, the first time the effects of a psychedelic were described in a scientific journal was in 1887, when a Texas doctor named John Raleigh Briggs wrote of his experience after eating peyote.[8] Ten years later, German pharmacologist and chemist Arthur Heffter isolated mescaline from the peyote cactus. It wasn't until the 1940s that scientists looked more seriously at psychedelics—mostly mescaline and LSD. Governments, too, examined these drugs, with German and U.S. militaries testing them on prisoners and agents as "truth drugs."[9] In the '50s, pioneering researchers and psychiatrists Humphry Osmond and Abram Hoffer began using LSD on patients suffering from alcohol use disorder in Saskatchewan, Canada, with much success.[10] (The two are considered to be the founders of psychedelic therapy, with Osmond responsible for coining the term *psychedelic*.)[11]

The unique effects of the "magic mushroom" were presented to North America for the first time in a 1957 photo essay in *Life* magazine that forever changed the community it documented. Written by R. Gordon Wasson, an amateur mycologist, "Seeking the Magic Mushroom" told readers of a "remote Mexican Indian village" where "vision-giving fungi" were held in divine regard and regularly consumed in congregational settings.[12] Psychologist Timothy Leary read the story, and in 1959 began lecturing at Harvard University's Department of Psychology. He joined forces with another psychology researcher, Richard Alpert (later known as Ram Dass), to create the Harvard Psilocybin Project. Through this, the two administered psilocybin to volunteer subjects and documented its effects on their consciousness—while consuming it themselves. Their work turned many American college students on to psychedelics, but Leary and Alpert's casual attitude toward scientific standards proved to be problematic. Around the same time, the media began to run with horrifying (but unverified) stories of "black market" LSD that caused birth defects, brain damage, and psychotic episodes.[13]

Seeds of fear had also been planted in 1962, when researcher Sidney Cohen expressed concern about the popularization of LSD and its nonmedical use.[14] While Cohen himself was an early proponent of LSD and concluded through his own work that, when administered in a medical setting, it was safe, he wrote a paper in 1962 warning fellow scientists of the dangers of improper LSD use when hospitalizations and accidents began to increase. (In a few cases, it was reported that people who took "acid" died while under the influence of the drug.) That same year, amendments to the Food, Drug, and Cosmetic Act made it so that scientists interested in studying LSD (or any pharmaceutical) had to establish the drug's efficacy before conducting their research. The new emphasis on rigorous clinical trial methods and study design significantly impeded their work on psychedelic psychotherapy.[15]

In the spring of 1963, Leary and Alpert were fired for administering psilocybin to undergraduate students off-campus after agreeing with the institution that they would only use graduate students as volunteers.[16] The end of the Harvard Psilocybin Project only furthered the narrative fueled by Cohen that psychedelics were dangerous. Being fired didn't stop Leary from having a profound influence on North American counterculture; at a music festival in San Francisco in January 1967, he famously uttered the words "Turn on, tune in, drop out," a slogan that would be printed on T-shirts, posters, and banners, and quickly became the unofficial slogan of the psychedelic counterculture.

While Leary and Alpert's work was not held in high regard by the scientific community, researchers like Czech psychiatrist Stanislav Grof, who, like Osmond and Hoffer, had had tremendous results with patients when combining psychedelics with psychotherapy, began to set a new bar for psychedelic research. Grof studied psychedelics in Czechoslovakia before relocating to the U.S. in 1967, where he became a research fellow and then a professor at Johns Hopkins University. In a 2014 NPR interview, he recounted the feeling at the time: "It was quite extraordinary... This was a tremendous deepening and acceleration of the psychotherapeutic process, and compared with the therapy in general, which mostly focuses on suppression of symptoms, here we had something that could actually get to the core of the problems."[17]

The War on Drugs

SOME PEOPLE WILL tell you that the prohibition of psychedelics began with former U.S. president Richard Nixon's War on Drugs and the "all-out offensive" on drug abuse he launched on June 17, 1971.[18] But though they went largely unenforced, the first laws in North America banning psychedelics were passed much earlier. LSD was first prohibited at the state level in California and Nevada in 1966, with New York following suit.[19] Despite the new law in California, LSD was used widely at outdoor concerts like the Trips Festival, a brainchild of novelist Ken Kesey, and the Monterey Pop Festival. Six months after the Golden State's law was passed, the Grateful Dead played the infamous Human Be-In in San Francisco's Golden Gate Park to observe the drug's criminalization, and to wave their collective middle finger at the establishment that wanted to take their drug of choice away.[20]

One progressive politician, Senator Robert (Bobby) Kennedy, didn't understand the speed with which the government had changed its mind on LSD, and issued a congressional probe into the matter.

"Why if [clinical LSD projects] were worthwhile six months ago, why aren't they worthwhile now? I think ... to some extent we have lost sight of the fact that it can be very, very helpful in our society if used properly," he said in a presentation to the group that would eventually become the Drug Enforcement Administration (DEA).[21] His interest in LSD research, it turns out, was personal: Kennedy's wife, Ethel, had received LSD treatment at Hollywood Hospital in New Westminster, British Columbia, an experimental private hospital run by physician J. Ross MacLean and Al Hubbard, a wealthy businessman and one of the first proponents of LSD treatment.

At the time, some of the most important psychedelic and psychology research was taking place in Canada. In Saskatchewan, work had started even earlier than it had in B.C. Home to the first socialist government and universal health-care program in North America, the province attracted experts like Dr. Osmond, who moved there to serve as a director of the Weyburn Mental Hospital in 1951. Together with Hoffer, he administered LSD to an estimated 2,000 patients. Until Hollywood Hospital closed in 1975, MacLean and Hubbard supervised more than 6,000 acid trips for patients who hoped to overcome alcohol use disorder, anxiety disorders, depression, and even marital discord.[22] Other notable patients there included the actor Cary Grant and the singer Andy Williams. (Coincidentally, I live in the neighborhood where the hospital was once situated. Today, a grocery store sits on the property, and while shopping for produce I often find myself wondering what patients at the hospital might have experienced.)

Kennedy's probe received little attention. Then, in October 1968, U.S. Congress passed the Staggers-Dodd Bill, which amended the Food, Drug, and Cosmetic Act to ban the personal possession of LSD at the federal level.[23] Two years later, on October 27, 1970, the Controlled Substances Act was signed into law, defining a scheduling system that classified drugs including LSD, magic mushrooms, MDMA, and even cannabis as having "no medical value" and a "high potential for abuse." This classification system changed the way psychedelics were viewed on a global level, and soon other nations followed suit. In Canada, where the Narcotic Control Act had come into force in 1961, enforcement increased substantially, particularly for offenses related to cannabis. (Canada eventually introduced its own drug schedule in 1996.) In the United Kingdom, the Misuse of Drugs Act 1971 set out classes of drugs similar to those used in America's Controlled Substances Act, while Australia introduced its own drug scheduling system in 1989.

With Nixon's proclamation of war, psychedelics were swiftly forced back into Pandora's box, at least from an academic standpoint, for several decades. When the Controlled Substances Act became law, the National Institute of Mental Health ceased to provide funding to researchers and universities, while the DEA no longer gave scientists the approval they needed to possess LSD for research. This brought all study of LSD and other psychedelics in the U.S. to an abrupt halt. Still, some researchers, most notably Alexander Shulgin, continued to work on psychedelics underground—with Shulgin introducing MDMA to therapists in the United States in 1976.[24]

The Post-Psychedelic Era

IN THE 1980S, vilifying mind-altering substances was commonplace in America—who can forget Nancy Reagan's "Just Say No" campaign, or the infamous PSA that likened a sizzling egg to a brain on drugs? These campaigns didn't stop the black market for psychedelics. Two underground chemists, Tim Scully and Nick Sand, would continue to synthesize acid—a legendary version of the drug endearingly referred to as Orange Sunshine—in massive quantities. They produced four million doses of the stuff before being busted. Sand decided to flee and spent the next twenty years in a clandestine lab in Canada, continuing his craft in defiance of the law. Throughout his life, he made nearly 14 kilograms of LSD and its analogues, about 140 million trips' worth.[25] (We'll hear from one of his former partners in chapter 2.)

The late 1980s and early 1990s saw a revival of interest in psychedelics, thanks to rave culture and alternative rock, as well as to cultural influencers like Terence McKenna. To help with research efforts, activist Rick Doblin founded the nonprofit Multidisciplinary Association for Psychedelic Studies in 1986, to raise funds and apply for the necessary approvals. The Heffter Research Institute was founded with a similar purpose in 1993. Human research was renewed after scientists challenged the FDA to treat hallucinogenic drug research the same way it treated research on other drugs. Some of the most noteworthy psychedelic research of the era was conducted on DMT by psychiatrist Rick Strassman. Psychedelic trials on humans picked up around the turn of the new millennium with studies from psychiatrist Charles Grob and psychologist Ralph Metzner, and the establishment in 1998 of the Beckley Foundation, a U.K.-based organization. It was founded by Amanda Feilding, Countess of Wemyss and March, and dedicated to the study of psychoactive substances and global drug-policy reform.

As researchers warmed to the idea of studying psychedelics again, so too did the establishment. In 2000, researchers at Johns Hopkins University were given regulatory approval to study psychedelics in healthy volunteers, and began by considering the meaning of mystical experiences occasioned by psilocybin. The groundbreaking 2006 study was the first of many on psilocybin to come out of the institution. (Where LSD was the psychedelic of choice among researchers in the 1960s, psilocybin emerged as the substance preferred by researchers of the current era, at least among the so-called "classic" psychedelics, for its shorter duration and less problematic history.) Throughout the 2000s, organizations like MAPS, Heffter, and Beckley, along with countless private donors, provided funding for studies that revisited some of the work carried out in the 1960s. More recent studies into psychedelics consider a broad range of potential applications, and in some cases take technologies like brain imaging into account. In addition, we're seeing more randomized, double-blind, placebo-controlled trials—the so-called gold standard of scientific evidence.

We have just barely scratched the surface of the science that has emerged since the War on Drugs began, and of the potential these long-used compounds have for a growing list of medical conditions—not to mention their ability to optimize thought and creativity among healthy populations. As we dive into the next seven chapters to discuss these compounds in greater depth through history, culture, research, expert testimony, and real-life accounts, I invite you to open your mind to the possibilities and put any preconceptions you might have about psychedelics on the proverbial shelf.

THE
CLASSIC
PSYCHEDELICS

Classic psychedelics include psilocybin, LSD, DMT, and mescaline.[1] While all psychedelics trigger altered states of consciousness, these compounds work by interacting with serotonin receptors known as 5-HT2 receptors, of which there are several subtypes distributed throughout the central nervous system and highly concentrated in the brain. The hormone serotonin is known for its role in stabilizing mood and promoting feelings of well-being. It also enables communication among brain cells. Classic hallucinogens target these receptors and act as agonists, which means they trigger physiological responses associated with serotonin when they come into contact with the receptor.

Classic psychedelics can be broken down further based on their structure: psilocybin, LSD, and DMT, like serotonin, are of the tryptamine class, while mescaline is a phenethylamine alkaloid. It is the stimulation of the 5-HT2A receptor that triggers the profound and potentially life-altering experiences brought on by classic psychedelics. (To test this, researchers blocked the receptor with another compound, a serotonin agonist. They found that when the receptor is blocked, these effects do not occur.)[2] Each compound can inspire wildly different experiences, and even consistent doses of the same drug in the same individual can elicit very distinct trips, as psychedelic journeys are largely influenced by one's biology, expectation, intention, and environment.

In the United States, Canada, the European Union, and the United Kingdom, classic psychedelics are controlled substances, meaning regulators have decided, rightly or wrongly, that they possess a high level of abuse potential and no medical benefit. As such, they are illegal to possess or sell unless for scientific or exempted medical purposes. While these drugs are increasingly being used for research purposes, they can and have been misused and can lead to harm. In rare cases, the anxiety or fear sparked by a bad trip can sometimes lead to self-harm and even accidental death. These instances serve as a powerful reminder that one *must* consider the who, what, when, where, why, and how of one's psychedelic experience, preferably well before consuming the substance in question.

Each of these substances can produce trips of varying length, depending on dose and method of administration. While the effects of psilocybin generally persist from four to six hours, LSD trips can last up to twelve hours. When smoked or injected, the effects of DMT are experienced almost immediately and can last thirty to forty-five minutes. However, when DMT is consumed in the form of ayahuasca, a potent sacred tea revered by several Indigenous communities in the western Amazon basin, its effects can be felt for four to six hours. Experiences with mescaline-containing cacti like peyote or San Pedro may last between nine and twelve hours or longer.

The specific effects of these substances vary and can in many ways overlap, while remaining unique from one another. All classic psychedelics have been known to inspire mystical experiences. One study describes this state as "feelings of unity and interconnectedness with all people and things, a sense of sacredness, feelings of peace and joy, a sense of transcending normal time and space, ineffability, and an intuitive belief that the experience is a source of objective truth about the nature of reality."[3] Findings in other studies show that, following these sorts of experiences in clinical settings, individuals report changes in behavior, values, and attitudes that may last well over a year.

1. Psilocybin

BEYOND MAGIC MUSHROOMS

Case Study
A Guided Trip to Overcome and
Integrate Childhood Trauma

In her thirties after several years of therapy, Eman Salem felt that she was finally ready to take what she perceived to be the next step in overcoming the trauma and abuse she had survived as a child: a guided experience with psilocybin mushrooms. She had heard great things about their potential to help, but given her inexperience with them, the idea terrified her. She recognized well in advance that to optimize her experience, she would have to prepare herself.

"As a survivor of abuse, there are a lot of things about the body that I just couldn't let go of," Salem says from her home in Vancouver when we connect on Zoom. Psychologically, she understood that she would be in an environment where she'd be cared for, but she anticipated discomfort. Her prep work revolved around an important question: "Can I create a safe environment for myself so that I can truly explore what it's like not to be anxious about my body, and not be anxious for my safety?" While integration (in short, the emotional work done after a psychedelic experience to make sense of and act on the lessons you received) often gets all the attention, Salem highlights the importance of the mental and emotional preparation that can help reduce anxiety and feelings of fear around an impending psychedelic trip.

To help mitigate some of her fear, Salem chose to work one-on-one with an experienced underground psilocybin practitioner in their dedicated environment, carefully suited to the first-time psilocybin user: decor was simple yet pleasing, a space she described as "smooth, so that it doesn't force anything onto your experience." After settling in with calm, ambient music, the guide led Salem through a ritual and helped establish her intention: that whatever might come through her experience, no matter how dark, would be for her healing. Then she consumed four grams of psilocybin mushrooms in the form of chocolates—well above an average dose.

"It was a very dark, painful trip. There wasn't laughing and cracking jokes . . . it was truly going into the depths and pulling out all my demons and facing them," she recalls, describing what it was like to come face-to-face with her depression and anxiety. Salem says she spent at least half of the experience lying down, and while it's tough for her to recall exactly what happened, she was able to work through multiple issues with her guide inside the container of the ceremony. While working with psilocybin, Salem was also able to experience an important revelation. After years of feeling ashamed of her body, she gave herself permission "to start showing up" exactly as herself.

"I think even though it may seem like I always did that, there was such a heaviness in the heart, because I was sad. I was sad all the time, and resentful all the time. I was very angry at the things that happened to me that I had no control over, especially as a child," she says. "One of the biggest things I struggled with is a lot of the abuse came from my family, who is also the most loving family. There was a moment where I met my parents as their child selves. It was child me who met them, and from a child to a child, you can't see that person as an abusive person or a narcissist, you just see them as a human being. You're like, 'What, another kid? Let's go play!'" she exclaims.

"I really did feel what it would be like to not have resentment towards them, and I cried for days about that, because I realized they were just human beings who did shit. In that trip, it all just crashed, and I didn't have to revisit those memories anymore. I was able to just see these children play."

Afterward, Salem made sense of her experience over the course of several integration sessions with her guide. Since then, she says, her life has seen a dramatic shift, and she's grateful for the bird's-eye view that the psilocybin trip has left her with.

"It's a stupid thing to ever suggest that if you take mushrooms, all of a sudden you're going to have no problems," she says. Yet Salem has experienced new levels of joy and elation since her trip, shedding fear about her queer identity, and embracing every facet of self-expression. She sees psilocybin mushrooms as one of many tools that she can use to look inward.

"I am so much bigger, so much more grand, so much more than I had ever allowed myself to feel," she says. "There is a whole other level of self-awareness."

How Psilocybin Works

WHILE LSD RECEIVED much attention from psychotherapists in the first wave of psychedelic research, psilocybin is the preferred substance among researchers today for a few reasons. One of the leading researchers on psychedelics, Dr. Robin Carhart-Harris, explains that there are a few factors at play, not the least of which is stigma.

"But it's not just that," says Carhart-Harris, head of the Neuroscape Psychedelics Division at the University of California, San Francisco, when we speak over Zoom. "We've done studies with psilocybin, and we've done some studies with LSD, and we've realized that psilocybin is just easier to manage. You can get great therapeutic outcomes with psilocybin, without the need to have a longer trip." Both psilocybin and LSD work in the same way, interacting with the 5-HT2A receptor, initiating "a cascade of processes that do different things," he says.

"This specific receptor is involved in plasticity, which basically means the ability for the system to change—to be shaped or molded." Psychedelics like psilocybin, he says, help people adjust their perspectives about themselves and the world—just as Eman Salem did when she came to a new relationship with her past. This is what the term *neuroplasticity* refers to: the brain's ability to modify, change, and adapt throughout life.

"If you couldn't enhance plasticity, people would be stuck, and they couldn't relearn," says Carhart-Harris. Some scientific research, he says, suggests that psychedelics also increase the excitability of the neurons that house the serotonin 2A receptors—that is, psychedelics make them more likely to transmit the messages that serotonin and other substances tell them to transmit. "In a sense, your receptive bandwidth has been broadened a bit, like going from terrestrial TV to satellite TV in the '90s."

There's also a hint that mushrooms may have helped our brains evolve. Carhart-Harris says recent science suggests that there's a link between the serotonin 2A receptor's signaling and the evolution of the human brain. Several systems in the human brain, including the default mode network, the part of the brain that is home to our ego, emotions, and memory,[1] are more developed than they are in other mammals. "Their expansion was at least in part triggered by signaling via the psychedelic serotonin 2A receptor," he says.

Some researchers, including ethnopharmacologist Dennis McKenna, believe the consumption of psilocybin mushrooms played a critical role in human evolution. While his brother Terence was known for profound psychedelic proclamations and powerful tripping advice, the quieter of the two McKenna brothers has committed most of his life to spreading the word in other ways, hosting retreats in South America and participating in seminars and conferences where he speaks about the inherent benefits of numerous psychedelic medicines, including mushrooms and ayahuasca.

Dennis and his brother are known for putting forth a hypothesis called the "stoned ape" theory, which suggests that the human brain evolved to the size it is today—nearly tripling in size in two million years—because early humans consumed psilocybin-containing mushrooms. Terence McKenna, who passed away in 2000, first described this theory in his 1992 book, *Food of the Gods*.

Touching on McKenna's theory, Carhart-Harris points out that he may very well have been on the right track, given the aforementioned study: "So, Terence McKenna ... put his focus on psychedelics. Had he put his focus on the receptor that psychedelics hijack, he would have, in a sense, struck gold."

While Carhart-Harris says it will likely be several years before psilocybin is fully endorsed by the medical system and permitted for use in a therapeutic setting, its illegality hasn't stopped an increasing number of people from turning to it. And with a growing number of regions in North America passing initiatives to permit its use, he's confident that it will soon be available to more than just clinical trial participants with treatment-resistant mental health diagnoses.

Administration, Dosing, and Effects of Psilocybin

PSILOCYBIN CAN BE ADMINISTERED in a few different ways. In casual home use and underground therapy sessions, it is most often consumed as dried mushrooms, which can be ground and mixed into chocolates, or brewed into a tea. (Most clinical trials utilize synthetic psilocybin.) While the exact psilocybin content of dried mushrooms will vary from batch to batch and from stem to cap, the rule of thumb is that 1 gram of dried mushrooms contains about 10 milligrams of psilocybin. A 1-gram dose of mushrooms or 10-milligram dose of psilocybin is considered low, but is not to be confused with a microdose (something I'll cover later in this book), which involves taking even smaller doses of psilocybin, sometimes as low as 0.1 or 0.25 milligrams. In comparison, the hero's dose that propelled Daniel Carcillo into healing (described on page 29) was roughly 5 grams of mushrooms, or 50 milligrams of psilocybin. Generally, the effects of psilocybin can last anywhere from four to six hours.

While its effects will vary depending on dose, mindset, setting, sensitivity, tolerance, mushroom variety, and a range of other factors, feelings of euphoria and enhanced senses can be expected after taking as little as 5 milligrams of psilocybin, or half a gram of dried mushrooms. Heavier perceptual distortions can be expected with 1.5 to 2 grams, and as the dose goes up, so too will the intensity of such changes to perception. Ego dissolution, or the feeling of losing one's subjective identity, can be experienced at even higher doses of 3 to 3.5 grams, while a heroic dose of 5 grams or more might lead to a complete (temporary) disconnection from this earthly dimension. While ego dissolution sounds scary, it promotes feelings of interconnectedness and oneness with the universe and is often part of a larger mystical experience. The spectrum of emotions one can expect to feel ranges from giddy, excited, and euphoric to sad, paranoid, and anxious. Many people report a feeling of deep connection to nature and the world around them. Side effects like nausea and upset stomach can sometimes occur.

Psilocybin Mushrooms: Early Use

YOU MAY HAVE only recently learned of the therapeutic potential of psilocybin mushrooms (of which there are more than 180 different species growing all over the world),[2] but human use of these powerful fungi is nothing new. In fact, some archaeologists suggest the mushroom iconography depicted in rock art found in Australia and Africa is symbolic of the early use of psychoactive mushrooms. Images in the Gwion Gwion rock paintings (previously referred to as the Bradshaw rock paintings) in Western Australia and Sandawe rock art in what is now Tanzania date all the way back to 10,000 BCE and contain depictions of humans with mushroom heads. According to a 2011 study, "extant Sandawe shamans testify that this depiction represents the subjective experience of a trance under the influence of magic mushrooms."[3] There is also evidence to suggest ancient civilizations such as Egypt, Rome, and Greece used psychedelic mushrooms for religious purposes—in the case of ancient Egypt, reserving their use strictly for royalty.[4]

Psychedelic fungi grow on every continent, and so, naturally, other places in the world also show evidence of the early use of magic mushrooms. Throughout Mexico and Central America, mushroom statues were erected between 100 and 1400 CE, and some in a region of central Guatemala possibly date even earlier, from around 500 BCE.[5] Spiritually revered, these mushrooms were referred to as *teonanácatl*, a word in the Nahuatl language used by the Maya, Aztec, and Toltec civilizations meaning "god mushroom" or "flesh of the gods." When Spanish colonizers arrived in what is now Mexico, they attempted to rid local communities of their traditions and practices involving the consumption of sacred mushrooms in ceremonial settings, which appeared to them as a ritual not unlike Holy Communion.[6]

The Consequences of Seeking the Magic Mushroom

DESPITE THE SPANISH ATTEMPT to put an end to the religious use of mushrooms, ceremonies continued in Mexico, but they were forced underground. Most North Americans weren't officially introduced to "magic" mushrooms until R. Gordon Wasson's seminal photo essay was published in *Life* magazine in 1957—the first publication to ever refer to them as such. "Before the Spanish Conquest, mushrooms were very important in public ceremonies," he wrote. "The Conquest put a sudden end to the public ceremonies. Private meetings, because of their intimacy and despite the harassment of the Inquisition, have survived to date."[7]

Wasson and his wife found themselves privileged to participate in a mushroom ceremony known as a *velada* in the Oaxaca town of Huautla de Jiménez, led by María Sabina, a Mazatec *curandera* or healer known as the "Priestess of Magic Mushrooms." By publishing photographs and writing about their mushroom experience in a national magazine, Wasson publicized not only the rite, but the region too. The result was a flood of tourists visiting the small town, with the shared goal of seeing the same visions and achieving the level of awakening described in the *Life* piece.

At first, the priestess welcomed these visitors, but when the village became overrun, its residents turned on Sabina, running her out of town and burning her house down. Later in life, she felt regret for introducing Wasson to the mushrooms, which she referred to as saint children: "From the moment the foreigners arrived to search for God, the saint children lost their purity," she said.[8] Today, as psychedelic plant medicines including psilocybin mushrooms and ayahuasca are becoming increasingly popular, Sabina's story serves as a stark reminder of what can happen when protocols are appropriated, and when the keepers of important cultural and religious rites are not given the respect or support they deserve. As modern medicine revives psychedelic potential, it is important to remember that some psychedelic plant compounds have been used medicinally, spiritually, and recreationally long before the randomized, controlled clinical trial was deemed the gold standard.

Mushrooms as Divine Teachers

"INDIGENOUS PEOPLES TALK about these things as plant teachers—we will make an exception for mushrooms, technically they're not plants—but I think the idea that they are teachers, that you can learn from them, is something that everyone can benefit from," Dennis McKenna told me in 2019, when I interviewed him for the online magazine *Inside the Jar*.[9] Mushrooms continue to be revered in this way among the Mazatec, an Indigenous group living in the Sierra Mazateca in the Mexican state of Oaxaca, not only as teachers but as divine beings that can awaken us to our own divinity. This is in sharp contrast to using mushrooms to "trip."

Anthropologist and historian Inti García Flores is Mazatec and lives in Huautla de Jiménez. He tells me in Spanish, over email, that because of the impact of Western culture, the mushroom ritual has suffered. He calls what happened to his community's ceremonial use of the mushroom "an incursion" that put a price on something that, prior to the 1940s and 1950s, was considered priceless.

"The fungus and the ritual stopped being something secret and only for Mazatecs when they made publications and research regarding ritual use of the mushroom, making it public in magazines and books that were published for Western people only," he says. "We as the Mazatec community did not know what they were doing, or what was happening in the West with our rituals around the fungus. They did not come to be cured with the fungus, as we do, but were attracted to have an experience. They carried out extractivism of knowledge, and they became badly informed about how or why we use this medicine. That is where the sacredness of the fungus began to be distorted." García Flores says that most who use *Psilocybe cubensis* have yet to learn how sacred it truly is.

"It implies a whole ritual for its ingestion ... this medicine is really to cure or fix something, not just to feel good and see beautiful things. The mushroom is a sentient being and has its own voice. It knows how to communicate." As part of this relationship, García Flores says, one must also consider the lessons mushrooms teach us about reciprocity.

"Here in the Sierra Mazateca, to be reciprocal with the fungus is to take care of the spaces where they sprout naturally," he says, although he notes there is lack of support for creating a protected natural area for them. García Flores says it would only be fair, given the immense wisdom and healing that they provide. When it comes to reciprocity for Huautla de Jiménez, he's looked closely at the needs that exist in the community and says that to avoid repeating the past, the Mazatec will continue to refuse interference from people outside of their town.

"Thanks to the fact that we as Mazatecs have resisted and continue to do so despite the onslaught of modernity, we continue to preserve our great culture that gives us strength and identity in the world."

While much of modern medicine tends to focus on psychedelics as a means of personal healing, Indigenous ways of knowing have existed for thousands of years and have a lot more to teach us about how they can be used.

Case Study
Overcoming Traumatic Brain Injury With Magic Mushrooms

After winning two Stanley Cups with the Chicago Blackhawks in three short years, National Hockey League player Daniel Carcillo was ready to hang up his skates for good. Post-concussion syndrome had begun to catch up with him, and in 2015, the thirty-year-old left winger stepped off the rink after his last official game. Despite being at the height of his hockey career, Carcillo found himself overwhelmed with the physical, mental, and emotional symptoms associated with traumatic brain injury (TBI): headaches, trouble sleeping, light sensitivity, slurred speech, anxiety, impulsivity, depression, and suicidal ideation. His best friend and former teammate,

Steve Montador, had suffered from the same symptoms before dying unexpectedly at the age of thirty-five. For Carcillo, the loss of his friend, followed quickly by his seventh diagnosed concussion, sealed the deal.

Even though Carcillo knew deep down this was the end of his hockey career, leaving his teammates and the role he'd played on the ice was a dramatic shift. "What they tell you is 'Come back when you are symptom-free,' and I was never symptom-free," he says when speaking to me on Zoom. "One of the hardest things as hockey players is that we identify too much with the hockey part, rather than who we are as people. It was really scary to make a decision to walk away from the one thing that I thought defined me as a person."

Carcillo began dedicating every spare moment he had to learning more about TBI, creating a foundation of his own to support and advocate for others suffering from the condition. He went down many roads in search of effective treatment and was duped into trying a few experimental and ineffective ones before being introduced to psilocybin mushrooms. Today, he looks back on that time with appreciation. "All of that was totally necessary to be able to be at the point where I am now, because now, I have evidence from the last eighteen months that I have structurally changed my brain."

The structural change he speaks of began with an invitation to participate in a mushroom ceremony on a farm, where he took a "hero's dose" of psilocybin mushrooms (generally 5 grams or more) that he says saved his life. For eighteen months after this initial experience, he took maintenance or "micro" doses of psilocybin to help integrate his larger journey. He also followed up with a few more higher-dose journeys. He credits this alternating protocol with changing his brain, after qEEG scans at six, twelve, and eighteen months revealed that his brain had "no abnormalities." Even so, Daniel says it's not the mushrooms that deserve all the glory.

"This definitely isn't a miracle drug," he notes. "It's a medicine that allows you to create good habits and then stay on those habits, but you have to do the work. [In bigger doses], it has the potential to change our perspective on our injury. A lot of TBI patients want to become the person that we were before the injury, but I'm trying to show people that you can actually get better."

What the Science Says About...

PSILOCYBIN FOR END-OF-LIFE DEPRESSION AND ANXIETY

WHILE THE IDEA of looking inward can be frightful to some, it is precisely the act of doing so that can spur changes in a person's perspective. In a double-blind, randomized, crossover trial published in 2016, researchers at Johns Hopkins University wanted to find out how a guided experience with psilocybin would affect levels of depression and anxiety in individuals with life-threatening cancer diagnoses.[10] A total of 51 participants received both a low dose of psilocybin (1 or 3 milligrams per 70 kilograms of body weight) and a high dose (22 or 30 milligrams per 70 kilograms of body weight) in two different sessions over the course of approximately five weeks, with preparation and integration sessions before and after.

Five weeks after the first session took place, 92 percent of participants showed reduced symptoms of depression and anxiety. After six months, 79 percent maintained a significant response to the treatment. Depression and anxiety were significantly decreased, while quality of life, life meaning, death acceptance, and optimism increased. The study also indicated that no serious adverse events took place as a result of administering psilocybin to the participants. Six-month results showed that 65 percent of participants experienced symptom remission of depression, and 57 percent experienced symptom remission of anxiety.

Researchers found that one measure that predicted enduring changes in the attitudes, mood, behavior, and spirituality of participants was the feeling of union with God or the divine, one of the typical effects of psilocybin—suggesting "that mystical-type experience per se has an important role apart from overall intensity of drug effect."

When Thomas Hartle, a 52-year-old Saskatoon resident with stage-four colon cancer, read the results of the study, he felt like they were too good to be true. "But when you suffer from anxiety, you really look for whatever sources of relief you can get," he tells me when I interview him for *Forbes*.[11] Hartle recruited the assistance of an organization named TheraPsil, a nonprofit that helps Canadians gain legal access to psilocybin. It took advantage of a subsection of the Controlled Drugs and Substances Act that allowed the health minister to grant exemptions for medical use on a case-by-case basis. So far, the organization has assisted dozens of Canadians, including terminally ill and clinically depressed patients, as well as doctors and therapists, in the application process. Without hesitation, he says the experiences he's had with psilocybin have changed his perspective on death and dying.

"What it's changed the most for me is that the unknown of what can happen after you die doesn't feel so unknown to me anymore. Most of how we define ourselves is our experiences and memories and things like that. In the psilocybin experience, my consciousness existed in ways that had absolutely nothing to do with anything in this life," he says. "To exist in another state that has nothing to do with my identity here, and to feel comfortable and serene in that state, tells me that it's possible to have some sort of continuation of consciousness that goes beyond our experience here."

PSILOCYBIN FOR
MAJOR DEPRESSIVE DISORDER

A RANDOMIZED CLINICAL TRIAL conducted by researchers at the Johns Hopkins University School of Medicine and published in 2021 considered how psilocybin-assisted psychotherapy might affect the severity of major depressive disorder among a small group of adults aged twenty-one to seventy-five who were not taking antidepressants.[12] Before their sessions, participants prepared with therapists for a total of eight hours, and were then administered psilocybin on two occasions, about two weeks apart, receiving a moderately high first dose (20 milligrams of psilocybin per 70 kilograms of body weight) and a higher second dose (30 milligrams per 70 kilograms). For context, the authors of *Buzzed: The Straight Facts About the Most Used and Abused Drugs From Alcohol to Ecstasy* describe a "typical" dose of psilocybin as 4 to 10 milligrams, or two to four mushrooms of the genus *Psilocybe cyanescens*.[13] It makes sense in this case that a higher dose was administered, as previous literature has shown that higher doses are more likely to lead to a mystical-type experience. During their psilocybin sessions, participants wore eyeshades and headphones and listened to a curated playlist of music. Follow-up therapy sessions were also held after these experiences.

The study authors note that, compared with ketamine, which has also been used for the treatment of major depressive disorder and has been shown to relieve the effects of depression for up to two weeks, psilocybin provided a longer period of relief of at least four weeks, with 71 percent of participants showing a positive response to treatment after that time. It may also have advantages over ketamine in its lower potential for misuse and fewer adverse effects. The authors write that the effect size, or the measure of magnitude of the treatment on participants in this study, was 2.5 times greater than that associated with psychotherapy alone, and more than 4.5 times greater than that associated with antidepressant drugs. As such, they go so far as to suggest that an intervention with psilocybin "may be more acceptable to patients than widely prescribed antidepressant medications that confer substantially more problematic effects." They also note that the single session or handful of sessions that psilocybin psychotherapy requires has a significant advantage over existing treatment options that require daily administration.

Another recent study directly compared psilocybin psychotherapy with the U.K.'s leading antidepressant, escitalopram (brands of which include Cipralex and Lexapro). The phase 2, double-blind, randomized controlled trial was designed by Robin Carhart-Harris, while serving as the head of the Centre for Psychedelic Research at Imperial College London. A total of fifty-nine participants with major depressive disorder were enrolled in the study and separated into two groups: one that would receive psilocybin and another that would receive the antidepressant. The first group received a dose of 25 milligrams of psilocybin on two different occasions, three weeks apart. They also took placebo tablets for six weeks to mimic the experience of taking an antidepressant. In the second group, participants were given small doses of psilocybin (1 milligram, an imperceptible dose) on two occasions, and took two three-week rounds of the SSRI at doses of 10 milligrams and 20 milligrams. Both groups received talk therapy in conjunction with their treatment.[14]

"We standardized the amount of psychological support that people received in the two groups," Carhart-Harris tells me when I reach him over Zoom to discuss the study. "The structure was consistent with the standard way of psychedelic therapy, involving preparation, supervision, and integration." Out of all the measures researchers looked at in this study, the only one that did *not* favor psilocybin was the primary outcome, defined as the change in self-reported depression scores from baseline (taken at the beginning of the study) to scores collected six weeks later, using the Quick Inventory of Depressive Symptomatology. Because of the primary outcome, the study authors indicate that psilocybin can only be described as "at least as effective" as the leading antidepressant. Among secondary outcomes, however, psilocybin was generally favored. These outcomes included changes to scores on additional scales, including the Beck Depression Inventory, and the Montgomery-Asberg Depression Rating Scale. Both groups saw reduced levels of depression, but a closer look reveals that the psilocybin group saw greater results in a shorter period, including improvements in ability to feel pleasure and express emotions, and increased feelings of well-being. Feelings of anxiety and suicidal ideation were also reduced significantly. According to Carhart-Harris, participants in both groups experienced the same overall number of side effects, but there were significantly fewer cases of emotional blunting, sexual dysfunction, dry mouth, drowsiness, and anxiety in the psilocybin group, where the most common side effect was a headache the day after a psilocybin dose. While the results of the trial may be a little confusing, he says the public should be encouraged about psychedelics in the treatment of mental illness, especially with plans for larger, longer trials in the future.

PSILOCYBIN
AND INCREASED OPENNESS

THE VALUE OF the mystical-type experience delivered by psilocybin cannot be overstated. One study by researchers from Johns Hopkins University School of Medicine looked specifically at the way an experience with psilocybin might affect five domains of personality, including neuroticism, extroversion, openness, agreeableness, and conscientiousness. This study was based on existing research that found that psilocybin produced "robust changes" in areas including perception, cognition, affect, and volition.[15] To look at the effects of psilocybin on these personality domains, the study authors considered data from two existing double-blind controlled studies of psilocybin, which they had conducted in 2006 and 2011.

Results showed that, as hypothesized, the level of openness among the healthy adult participants increased significantly following their psilocybin experience. Also consistent with the authors' predictions, having a mystical experience was correlated with increases in openness. At a one-year follow-up, participants who'd had what researchers defined as "complete" mystical experiences—that is, those who scored over 60 percent in a states-of-consciousness questionnaire measuring unity, transcendence of time and space, ineffability and paradoxicality, sacredness, noetic quality, and positive mood—had slightly lower levels of openness than they'd had immediately following their psilocybin session, but levels were still much higher than at their initial screening. Follow-up sessions with those who did not have complete mystical experiences as defined by researchers revealed that they had levels of openness that were "nearly identical" to those that were measured during their screening and immediately after their sessions. These findings suggest that lasting change to core personality traits is possible with psilocybin, though, as always, the study's authors stress that replicating these results is important.

Case Study
A Self-Guided Journey Brings Gender Identity Relief

While the administration of psilocybin for research purposes almost always occurs in a clinical setting, the reality is most people who take psilocybin do so in environments that do not resemble a hospital or doctor's office. When Ivy Astrix, a trans woman who at the time had yet to reveal her gender identity to the world, decided to take 6 grams of mushrooms, she took them by herself in an environment she felt comfortable in: the purpose-built "trip room" of a friend's farmhouse where she wouldn't be disturbed by the noise of the city. While she had experimented with microdoses, this would be her first serious psychedelic experience. To prepare, she read descriptions of people's trips on the internet and spoke with several friends about some of their psychedelic experiences, but even with that knowledge, she wasn't sure what to expect.

"I had a broad expectation, but no idea of what would actually happen," she recalls. Astrix was in the midst of immense life change: she'd just left a tech job of ten years for a role in Canada's new cannabis industry, and had moved to a new city after undergoing gallbladder surgery. She was also grappling with feelings of gender dysphoria, feelings she'd struggled with since she was fourteen, and was unsure if and how she might reveal her true self to the world. Taking the mushrooms was her way of looking inward to assess whether these new achievements were truly meant to be part of her path, and how life might be altered if she stepped into herself more fully. "Even though I had this great job, I really felt bad sometimes," she says, noting that there were times she considered suicide. "I had broken free of a job that had me feeling like I was not living up to my full potential, but something always felt wrong presenting as male."

The trip, Astrix says, stirred up a feeling in her that she should "do something" about the feelings she had, rather than just let them be. In her line of sight, she'd arranged a makeshift altar with feminine imagery, and she'd prepared a playlist to match, chock-full of favorite musicians. She experienced classic psychedelic symptoms like seeing light tracers and powerful, kaleidoscopic visuals, but the most profound effects were the ones that prompted her to change her thinking about her gender identity and how she chose to present herself to the world. One of the biggest positive outcomes of the trip was the understanding she gained of her anxiety, especially around other people.

"So much of my social anxiety was wrapped up in gender dysphoria," she says. Astrix also experienced ego dissolution as part of her trip, something she had never felt before.

"The biggest revelation was 'If you have nearly every other aspect of your life at this top level, why is this not dealt with? Are you not doing a disservice to yourself at this point?'" she says. Importantly, Astrix felt supported by her community in the idea of coming out as trans. She was overwhelmed by glimpses into the future that showed her having impact in the trans community and the world at large, and by the feeling of connection she felt to her femininity.

"Being out publicly has been really good for me. Completely shifting gender roles really put me at ease, and solved a lot of my anxiety," she says. "It puts me at peace with myself."

PSILOCYBIN
FOR OCD

WHILE ANECDOTAL REPORTS from some people with obsessive-compulsive disorder (OCD) have suggested that psilocybin may be useful in treating the condition, there hasn't been much science to back it up. In the early 2000s, researchers at the University of Arizona set out to change that with a small study using just nine participants.[16] The authors note in its introduction that while SSRIs are thought to be the most effective treatment for OCD, they generally reduce symptoms by only 30 to 50 percent, and it's estimated between 40 and 60 percent of people who are treated for OCD will fail to respond. All the subjects involved in this study fit into that category.

Each participant was administered psilocybin on several occasions at different doses per kilogram of body weight, including a very low dose of 25 micrograms, a low dose of 100 micrograms, a medium dose of 200 micrograms, and a high dose of 300 micrograms. During their eight-hour sessions, they listened to music through headphones and wore eyeshades. Following their sessions, researchers used a variety of tests to measure the effects of the psilocybin experiences. Only six of the nine participants remained in the proof-of-concept, phase 1 trial long enough to take all four doses, with all nine receiving the low dose, and seven receiving the very low dose and medium dose. After the first dose, two participants quit the trial because of discomfort around hospitalization. Measurements taken up to twenty-four hours after each session revealed that almost 90 percent of subjects maintained a 25 percent or greater decrease in their symptoms, while two thirds maintained a 50 percent or greater decrease in their symptoms following at least one of the doses. Two of the participants reported symptom improvement lasting up to a week after being administered psilocybin, and one even achieved full remission according to a six-month follow-up.

Based on the small study, researchers concluded that psilocybin is a safe and well-tolerated substance when administered in a supportive "clinical" environment—though I find that word choice interesting, given the reason two of the nine participants dropped out of the trial: discomfort with hospitalization. This is an important thing to consider, because while a clinical setting might be the safest option in the eyes of a physician, the sterile environment may not be comfortable for people who otherwise qualify for such trial work.

PSILOCYBIN FOR SMOKING CESSATION

AN OPEN-LABEL PILOT STUDY conducted by researchers at Johns Hopkins University published in 2017 revealed psilocybin's potential to help people quit smoking cigarettes, a habit that causes more than six million deaths per year globally. Even the most effective existing smoking-cessation medications demonstrate less than 31 percent abstinence one year after treatment. A total of fifteen smokers took part in the study, each smoking an average of nineteen cigarettes a day, for an average of thirty-one years. For four weeks prior to being administered psilocybin, they took part in psychotherapy that combined cognitive behavioral therapy, mindfulness, and guided imagery. At week five, at the time of the intended quit date of those taking part in the trial, they were administered a dose of psilocybin classified as moderate (20 milligrams of psilocybin per 70 kilograms of body weight). Two weeks later, they were given another, slightly higher dose. An optional third experience with psilocybin was made available at week thirteen of the study.

A follow-up revealed that one year after the treatment, ten participants were confirmed to be smoking abstinent, with eight participants confirming they had not smoked a single cigarette since the study's target quit date. Unlike existing treatment options for smoking cessation, the treatment used in this study found 60 percent were able to abstain from smoking for up to one year following its administration.[17]

Recently, Johns Hopkins University was awarded a grant from the National Institute on Drug Abuse to conduct a three-year study focusing on psilocybin for tobacco addiction. It is the first federal grant given to investigate the therapeutic effects of a psychedelic in fifty years.

PSILOCYBIN
FOR ALCOHOL USE DISORDER

WHILE LSD OFTEN gets the most attention for its use in research around alcohol use disorder, a study published in 2018 considered how effective psilocybin might be at treating the same condition, presenting the case reports of three participants from a double-blind, randomized, placebo-controlled trial. Over the course of twelve weeks, participants received psychotherapy, and were given psilocybin during two of the sessions.

One of the subjects in the study, Mark, a young white man in his twenties, was a binge drinker who, on drinking days, would consume an average of twenty-two alcoholic beverages. He had attended Alcoholics Anonymous and tried treatment, but neither had worked. During his second psilocybin session, he said he was confronted by the different ways his drinking was harmful to himself and those around him. These feelings were followed by overwhelming joy at the thought of "being given a new slate." Mark remained abstinent from alcohol and opted for a third psilocybin session, where he was able to deal with feelings of disappointment, regret, shame, and unworthiness, as well as "eureka moments" that left him feeling calm and reassured when the session ended. The study's authors report that two years after his enrollment in the study, he remained abstinent.

Another subject, Rob, was a Black man in his forties who had grown up witnessing the harms of alcoholism, eventually losing his father to complications of the condition. He began drinking heavily in college, but after his father's death he became increasingly concerned about how alcohol would affect his health. His experience with psilocybin was in stark contrast to Mark's: he suffered nausea and abdominal pain and felt as though he might vomit. Sitting upright, he resisted the effects of the psilocybin for as long as he could, spitting into a bucket to rid his body of feelings of shame, resentment, anger, and fear. The next day, he reported that he'd felt the presence of his father. Later, Rob would describe the session to researchers: "Nothing ever felt worse than those two hours," he told them. He didn't participate in the second or third psilocybin sessions, but even after the wildly unpleasant experience, Rob reported feeling more forgiving of himself. He continued with the psychotherapy element of the study, and at a follow-up session conducted more than a year after the study began, he reported that he had remained abstinent.

The third subject presented in the study, Lisa, was a Latin-American woman in her fifties. As with Rob, alcoholism was part of her family's history. Lisa developed problem drinking around the age of thirty, often drinking alone and being overcome with feelings of guilt and shame. Like Mark, she had attended AA meetings and attempted treatment, but to no avail. During her first psilocybin session, Lisa had a conversation with God about her drinking and controlling nature. She reported improved mood and a decrease in self-critical thinking, and though she opted not to commit to complete abstinence, she did begin to drink much less. Lisa's second session with a higher dose of psilocybin put her in a confused and chaotic state of thought before she encountered overwhelming feelings of sadness. After surrendering control, she was overcome with feelings of peace and heard a voice tell her, "You are a perfect creation of the universe." This same voice asked Lisa over and over if she believed it, and in the end, her self-doubt and criticism were replaced by a state of profound self-acceptance. She later told researchers that after the second session, all critical self-thought had been pushed from her mind, and alcohol had almost no appeal to her anymore.

While the researchers note that each of these cases is different, they point out that regardless of whether a participant experiences a classic mystical or peak-psychedelic experience, psilocybin sessions "evoke material that is personally meaningful, with content that is uniquely relevant to each individual participant."[18]

2. LSD

THE DRUG THAT
ELEVATED A GENERATION

Case Study
Microdosing Leads
to Leveling Up

Paul Austin was first turned on to the idea of microdosing while listening to an episode of *The Tim Ferriss Show* featuring James Fadiman, a writer and pioneer of psychedelic research often referred to as "the father of microdosing." It was 2015, and Austin was living in Thailand and building his first tech start-up, an online coaching business and platform for English language teachers. He had taken LSD a few times before in his life, and the podcast episode reminded him of the warm glow he had experienced after those acid trips. Based on what he had heard, microdosing with LSD could give him the opportunity to reengage with that feeling without undergoing a ten- or twelve-hour trip, and so he decided to follow Fadiman's microdosing protocol as an experiment. From July 2015 to January 2016, Austin took a tiny dose of LSD twice a week.

"It was usually anywhere from 10 micrograms to 25 micrograms, so in some cases more of a mini dose than a microdose, where it was slightly perceptible but not overwhelming by any stretch of the imagination," he says today. "Since then, I've experimented with microdosing mushrooms, San Pedro, and iboga, but LSD has always been my favorite way to microdose."

While the afterglow feeling was what initially motivated him to try microdosing, the practice revealed two core intentions or guiding principles to Austin that encouraged him to continue.

"The first intention was to connect more with people, to ease social anxiety, and to reduce, if not eliminate, alcohol use," he says. On nights out, Austin would opt to microdose LSD instead of throwing back cocktails with his friends.

"I'd been in a fraternity in college and drank quite regularly, but when I graduated, I was getting more and more onto the personal-development path, and thought alcohol was really destructive. A lot of my friends were still drinking and going out in these entrepreneurial circles in Chiang Mai, and I thought, 'How cool would it be to do something like LSD instead of alcohol?' "

Austin's secondary intention had to do with tapping into states of creative flow: "Oftentimes, as an entrepreneur, there's a lot of resistance or procrastination or friction in terms of getting that creative engine going, and so I was looking to microdose with LSD to help with the ideation phase of building a business," he says. On microdosing days, which happened every fourth day, Austin was able to drop into states of total focus more easily, with less procrastination or internal friction.

While microdosing LSD, Austin founded Third Wave, an online platform and academy offering education and courses for those interested in learning more about psychedelics, with everything from microdosing guides to compound-specific primers. He also offers one-on-one microdosing coaching, a fact that inspired *Rolling Stone* to dub him "the world's first online LSD microdosing coach" in 2017.[1]

Reflecting on his first experience back in 2015, Austin says when it came to social anxiety and alcohol consumption, microdosing worked: "I was able to connect more with folks, to be more open instead of more guarded and in my head," he observes. "For that specific thing, it was very helpful." But when it came to Austin's goal of achieving better creative flow, microdosing was "almost too helpful." While microdoses of LSD can certainly help to achieve a flow state, he says there's an important distinction between that and mania.

"What I noticed with microdosing is that it was certainly helpful, but because I had done it twice a week for seven months, towards the end of that period, it started to burn me out a little bit," he notes. "I was in a more manic state because there was so much energy moving through... I became a little too open, a little less focused than I would have liked to have been."

Austin decided to stop microdosing to give his body and mind an opportunity to "reset," and help him gain a sense of how the protocol was helpful. In the grand scheme of things, he says, microdosing with LSD allowed him to bring ideas and ways of thinking to the forefront that modern society doesn't necessarily encourage.

"In the industrial period, all the drugs that we used were really focused on convergent thinking and getting shit done, like caffeine, tobacco, and stimulants. Now, these new substances that we're using, particularly cannabis and psychedelics, are more focused on creativity and the divergent thinking process," he says. "What I noticed with LSD is it often helped to tie together disparate ideas into something cohesive."

Microdosing, Austin says, has been extremely relevant to what he's been able to build in the psychedelic sphere, but more than that, it has represented a new paradigm: "This isn't just about the research. It's really an archaic revival of these medicines that we've been using for thousands of years."

How LSD Works

LIKE PSILOCYBIN, LSD is a classic psychedelic and a tryptamine that interacts with serotonin receptors. These receptors respond to chemical messengers that help cells in the brain communicate with one another. A federally funded study published in 2017 revealed more details about how LSD binds to the receptors on a cell.[2] Using X-ray crystallography, researchers at the University of North Carolina School of Medicine led by Dr. Bryan Roth determined that when LSD binds with a receptor, the receptor creates a sort of "lid" over the LSD molecule that keeps the LSD attached for longer, something researchers said could be an explanation for the drug's long-lasting effects.

"LSD takes a long time to get onto the receptor, and then once it's on, it doesn't come off," said Roth in an interview with the UNC School of Medicine newsroom about the results of the study.[3] "And the reason is this lid."

Administration, Dosing, and Effects of LSD

LSD IS ADMINISTERED orally, most often via "tabs" on perforated blotter paper to which a liquid solution containing the drug has been applied. An LSD trip can last an exceptionally long time, sometimes twice as long as the average magic mushroom trip, and with an exponentially smaller dose. (Acid is measured in micrograms, or millionths of a gram, rather than in milligrams, or thousandths of a gram.)

As with any other drug, dosing is subjective and will vary depending on several factors, but generally, a "normal" recreational dose is between 100 and 150 micrograms. Microdoses of acid, like the ones Paul Austin took, are about one tenth of that dose, closer to 10 micrograms.

LSD can be predictable in that the more you take, the more intense you can expect the experience to be, but in many other ways it can be very unpredictable. While the effects of psilocybin can come on more slowly, taking a tab of acid can feel like flipping a light switch. Rather than a gradual onset, your senses are not only suddenly heightened, but also trading roles. (Synesthesia, the phenomenon of seeing sounds or hearing colors, is often reported with LSD.) It's common to experience visual hallucinations, though they aren't often as frightening as popular culture would have you believe. Still, seeing furniture begin to move before your eyes, or feeling a row of invisible ants crawling up your leg, might create feelings of fear and anxiety. (This is why factors like mindset and setting are so important—being in a safe, familiar, and controlled environment can help prevent hallucination-related meltdowns.) The heightened colors and sounds often lead users to feelings of euphoria and awe at the world, of bliss and boundlessness, and sometimes to a mystical experience.

LSD is quite stimulating and is known to disrupt sleep. People under the influence of LSD may feel energetic, empathetic, and excited, but they may also feel overwhelmed, confused, or panicked. Physical symptoms can include sweating, increased heart rate, and increased body temperature. Some people who have used LSD describe an afterglow, a period following their trip in which life feels lighter, brighter, and generally positive.

The Origins of LSD

UNLIKE MAGIC MUSHROOMS, LSD is one of three psychedelic drugs covered in this book that were born not in nature but in a laboratory. The drug is known by many names, including acid, blotter, Lucy, and Alice. Its effects on humanity have been nothing short of revolutionary.

After graduating from the University of Zurich in 1929 with a doctorate in medicinal chemistry, chemist Albert Hofmann was hired by Sandoz Pharmaceuticals and tasked with synthesizing compounds found in medicinal plants. Hofmann was eager to study ergot, a fungus that grows on rye and similar grains, to create a circulatory and respiratory stimulant based on ergot's known capacity to constrict blood vessels and muscles. Ergot had historically been used medicinally for excessive bleeding, though only in small doses. Here's the thing with ergot: if not dosed carefully, it can be incredibly poisonous. If consumed in excess—say, through diseased grains like rye—it can lead to long-term effects of poisoning known as ergotism, which can cause convulsions, hallucinations, and even the loss of limbs to gangrene.[4] In 1918, scientists at Sandoz had isolated ergotamine from ergot, and found the alkaloid made for safer and more reliable dosing than the toxic fungus. It was eventually sold under the name Gynergen, as a treatment for migraines and bleeding. After the isolation of ergotamine, scientists at Sandoz gave up on studying it.

When Hofmann took on the complex ergot fungus in the lab, Arthur Stoll, his superior who had isolated ergotamine over a decade earlier, cautioned him: "I must warn you of the difficulties you face in working with ergot alkaloids," he told Hofmann. "These are exceedingly sensitive, easily decomposed substances, less stable than any of the compounds you have investigated... But you are welcome to try."[5] Around the same time

Hofmann picked up work on ergot at Sandoz, scientists at the Rockefeller Institute of New York isolated the common nucleus of all active compounds in ergot and called the chemical "lysergic acid." Hofmann began synthesizing lysergic acid and combined it with derivatives of ammonia (amines) to create twenty-five different lysergic acid compounds. The final one, a mix of lysergic acid and an amine called diethylamide, was modeled on an existing stimulant with similar properties called Coramine, and eventually became the most popular of his creations—though certainly not as the treatment for respiratory and circulatory issues he'd hoped it would be. Three other drugs synthesized by Hofmann during this time would prove to have medical value: Hydergine, to improve cognitive function in patients with dementia; Dihydergot, to treat migraine; and Methergine, used to stop bleeding in childbirth.

Lab testing revealed that the psychedelic compound known as LSD-25, or lysergic acid diethylamide, caused high levels of excitement and restlessness in animal subjects, but it didn't seem to possess any of the medical qualities Hofmann was looking for. "The new substance ... aroused no special interest in our pharmacologists and physicians; testing was therefore discontinued," Hofmann wrote in his 1980 book *LSD: My Problem Child*. "For the next five years, nothing more was heard of the substance LSD-25."[6]

The First Acid Trip

DESPITE ABANDONING his study of LSD because of its apparent lack of medicinal properties, Hofmann often wondered about unknown effects of the compound, describing his curiosity as "the feeling that this substance could possess properties other than those established in the first investigations."[7]

In 1943, he revisited the experimental substance and resynthesized it. In a subsequent report written to Stoll, he described the strange sensations that overcame him after accidentally absorbing some of the compound through his fingertips: "Last Friday, April 16, 1943, I was forced to interrupt my work in the laboratory in the middle of the afternoon and proceed home, being affected by a remarkable restlessness, combined with a slight dizziness. At home I lay down and sank into a not unpleasant intoxicated-like condition, characterized by an extremely stimulated imagination. In a dreamlike state, with eyes closed (I found the daylight to be unpleasantly glaring), I perceived an uninterrupted stream of fantastic pictures, extraordinary shapes with intense, kaleidoscopic play of colors. After some two hours this condition faded away."[5]

Three days later, in the first intentional acid trip ever, Hofmann decided to dose himself with what seemed like an incredibly small amount of the mysterious compound: just 250 micrograms, diluted in water. Active doses of other compounds were often a thousand times more potent, so he expected that nothing would happen. He took the dose at 4:20 in the afternoon. By 5 p.m., the trip was underway, and soon Hofmann became so disoriented that he was forced to ride his bicycle home from the lab accompanied by his assistant, but not before writing one quick entry in his lab journal: "17:00: Beginning dizziness, feeling of anxiety, visual distortions, symptoms of paralysis, desire to laugh."[8]

Once home, Hofmann drank a glass of milk in hopes that it might help quell the effects he was experiencing, and over the course of the evening, he consumed nearly half a gallon of the stuff, to no avail. A journal entry made two days later, recounting the evening, read: "Home by bicycle. From 18:00–20:00 most severe crisis." In LSD: My Problem Child, he describes a terrifying scene in which "familiar objects and pieces of furniture assumed grotesque, threatening forms." A neighbor who brought Hofmann more milk was "an insidious witch with a colored mask."

Today, we know that, generally, people return from trips involving even frighteningly large doses of acid with their minds intact—one report found that a fifteen-year-old girl with bipolar disorder who took 1,100 micrograms of LSD at a music festival not only returned to her normal human experience, but relieved her bipolar symptoms. A whole twenty years later, the symptoms of her disorder had not returned.[9] But Hofmann was the guinea pig, riding the acid wheel before anyone else and rightfully wondering whether the experience was going to leave him permanently brain-damaged. A doctor finally arrived to assess him and found nothing wrong with him except for a set of very dilated pupils. At this point, the chemist was already coming out of his self-inflicted state of terror and found himself returning to reality: "The horror softened," he wrote, "and gave way to a feeling of good fortune and gratitude ... and I became more confident that the danger of insanity was conclusively past." It was at this point Hofmann could finally relax into the parts of the acid trip that are so revered, including kaleidoscopic visuals, vivid pictures in the mind, and synesthesia.

The next morning, Hofmann awoke feeling refreshed, with a renewed sense of well-being. To his knowledge, no other substance "evoked such profound psychic effects in such extremely low doses." Just hours after his self-experiment, Hofmann concluded that this new compound would be in demand among a wide variety of medical specialists. This turned out to be true: in 1947, Sandoz introduced LSD as a commercially available psychiatric medication under the name Delysid. A handbook on the drug printed in 1964 suggests it for three potential indications: in patients with psycho-neuroses and/or psychoses, and in "normal" patients in con-junction with psychopharmacology, with the idea that it could give psychiatrists "insight into the world of ideas and sensations of mental patients."[10] What Hofmann did not predict was that LSD-25 was about to become one of the most famous drugs of the twentieth century.

The First Wave:
Early Cultural Acceptance

AFTER HOFMANN DISCOVERED LSD's effects in 1943, scien-tists studied it first as a psychotomimetic (a drug that produces symptoms that mimic psychosis). They were interested in its effects in humans because they believed it would help them better understand psychotic diseases, such as schizophrenia. At this time, only the psychedelic substances mescaline and hashish, a form of pressed cannabis, had been studied in this way by psychiatrists. American doctors took an interest in the drug when Sandoz, believing it had clinical applications, began sending them free samples in 1949, with psychiatrist Sidney Cohen chief among them. He first mentioned LSD in his research in 1953, and eventually took it himself in 1955. Though he anticipated feelings of paranoia, he wrote in a report after the experience that "the problems and strivings, the worries, and frustrations of everyday life vanished; in their place was a majestic, sunlit, heavenly inner quietude ... I seemed to have finally arrived at the contemplation of eternal truth."[11]

In the U.S., Cohen and psychologist Betty Eisner explored LSD's efficacy in psychotherapy settings as a potential cure for alcoholism and a spark for creativity. They consulted with Al Hubbard, a charismatic, wealthy individual who was a proponent of LSD in psychotherapy in Canada. Hubbard was the cofounder of Hollywood Hospital, the world's longest-running psychedelic clinic, located in New Westminster, Canada, where he and Dr. J. Ross MacLean had begun administering LSD for alcoholism in 1957.[12] By 1959, many believed LSD was a "miracle cure" for the disease.[13] (Even the cofounder of Alcoholics Anonymous, Bill Wilson, pitched the therapeutic use of acid to fellow AA board members. They failed to see its treatment potential.)

The tail end of the 1950s marked a shift in research, and psychiatrists like Oscar Janiger began giving LSD to artists and creatives with the hypothesis that it would spur creativity. Around this time, Cohen noticed that many researchers weren't being cautious in their administration of the drug, with some even hosting parties where all attendees were encouraged, if not obligated, to take acid. In 1962, he published a paper warning other scientists that misuse of the drug would likely hinder research efforts. While Cohen wrote that the drug was safe, he made it clear it should only be administered in medical settings. Once one of the greatest academic supporters of LSD, Cohen lost interest in researching it, citing concerns that drug research and pseudoscience were starting to overlap, and he severed his working relationships with Hubbard and Eisner. The same year, Timothy Leary was introduced to LSD, and after the so-called Harvard drug scandal in 1963, in which he and his colleague Richard Alpert were fired for giving psychedelics to undergraduate students, LSD fell swiftly out of favor in the media. At the same time, it thrived in a counterculture that rejected authority and defied government.

Case Study
Becoming a
Psychedelic Chemist

Twenty-year-old Peter Van der Heyden was living in a squat in Leiden, Holland, enrolled in a university geology program but preoccupied with the fun he was having with a group of travelers from North America. It was 1972, and the narrative around LSD had shifted significantly since the previous decade: fear and paranoia about its risks had taken the place of any excitement or hope for its potential. With Timothy Leary's infamy and countless news stories about acid trips gone wrong, LSD was perceived by most as a dangerous, if not potentially deadly, substance. Van der Heyden had parked himself in the camp of young people who weren't interested in touching it because of its alleged risks.

"I didn't have a clue about what any of these things were, except that I thought they made you jump out of buildings," he says, referring to the sensationalized stories his parents had read about people who thought the drug could make them fly. (In 1969, it was widely reported that Diane Linkletter, daughter of TV personality Art Linkletter, had jumped out of her kitchen window after an acid trip. While she did jump to her death, the connection to LSD has since been debunked.)[14]

"I really wasn't interested in them. In fact, I was afraid of them," Van der Heyden recalls. When one of his new friends suggested he take LSD for the first time, he thought, "'He doesn't look like he's crazy. He's not acting weird. He's not dangerous. In fact, he's very friendly, very approachable, and very convincing.' I thought that maybe I'd been told some lies about this, and quickly, I confirmed that," Van der Heyden says of his change of heart. "I allowed myself to be persuaded to try a legendary form of LSD known as Orange Sunshine, and that changed my life. The influence of that first trip, it's still changing my life, and it's still the path that I'm on."

The experience itself was far from what he had imagined. So intrigued was Van der Heyden by this particular type of LSD—Orange Sunshine was an iconic variety characterized by its purity[15]—his instinct was to meet the person who had made it. "This was an intention of mine for about three days. I walked around and said, 'I want to meet the person who did this.'" Eventually, "life would take over," and Van der Heyden forgot he had ever had the idea.

Several years later in Canada, his aim would come to fruition: by complete chance, he met Nick Sand, coproducer of the famed Orange Sunshine. Van der Heyden promptly joined forces with Sand to go underground and make LSD. Before meeting Sand, he'd dabbled in psychedelic chemistry in a lab he ran at a local university, but he'd never imagined working at the scale Sand did.

"He said, 'If you start working with me, I'll teach you to do this with shovels and wheelbarrows, rather than small containers,'" Van der Heyden says. "Particularly with LSD, Nick was on a mission to supply the world." After each batch, he and Sand would stare at their creation and say, "May this benefit all of humanity."

Van der Heyden continued to work with Sand, producing LSD and other psychedelics in a lab in Sand's home until the massive operation was busted in 1996. Sand, who was already in trouble with officials in Canada and the U.S., was extradited and served time, while Van der Heyden was let off. He returned to geology for two decades, and today sees it as a "brief" interruption in his career in psychedelics. In 2017, thinking he was on the edge of retirement, he attended a psychedelic science conference in Oakland, California, and was reunited with several former friends, who are now colleagues. He learned that although psychedelic research was picking up, a reliable source of quality compounds was hard for researchers to come by. Within a few years, Van der Heyden decided against retirement and dived back into psychedelic chemistry—legally, this time—to create his own company and synthesize psychedelics for use in scientific research and clinical trials.

A Lifetime of Fascination With the Mystical Experience

AFTER PSYCHEDELIC RESEARCH was brought to a standstill, no woman proved to be more committed to the pursuit of research on LSD than Amanda Feilding. The Countess of Wemyss and March was an early cultural adopter of LSD who first took the drug in 1965. Six months into her experimentation with acid, a man she didn't trust spiked her coffee with thousands of micrograms of LSD.

"That was a very, very bad experience to have on psychedelics," recalls the countess (who also goes by Lady Neidpath), speaking with me from her home in Oxford. Had she not taken the next three months to recuperate in a hut in Beckley, England, she "would have decided never to touch another psychedelic again." But she did, and during her first experience back on the scene, at a party played by Indian sitarist Ravi Shankar, she was introduced to a Dutch librarian named Bart Huges.

Feilding and Huges, who went to medical school but said later in life he was refused a degree because he was an advocate of cannabis use, proceeded to fall in love, experimenting with psychedelics and documenting their experiences as they went, kicking off Feilding's lifelong commitment to psychedelic self-study. The ideas she and Huges promoted weren't always well received by the academic or medical communities—they were also advocates of trepanning, which involves boring a hole in one's skull for the purposes of so-called consciousness expansion, an experiment Feilding carried out on herself with a dentist's drill in 1970. But a few of Feilding's early instincts about LSD would eventually prove to be true.

Pushing for the Second Wave of Research

TWENTY-SEVEN YEARS after the start of the War on Drugs and more than thirty years since she'd first committed to studying LSD and other methods of consciousness expansion, Feilding created the Beckley Foundation, named after the property she still lives on today, to pursue psychedelic research and inspire changes in global drug policy.

"It's essential that drug policy be based on scientific evidence... but as a woman without letters after my name, it was very difficult to change global policy and open the doors to scientific research. I'd been devoted to searching for the benefits of psychedelics in a scientific way since 1966, and I realize now, it very much felt like Sisyphus pushing a rock up a cliff face," she says. This didn't get in her way, and in 1998, she launched her foundation.

Though most psychedelic research had dried up by this time because of restrictive policies across most of Europe and North America, Feilding was successful in bringing some of the world's top psychedelic experts together, including Albert Hofmann, to discuss global drug policy and how they might go about studying psychedelics once again.

"I've been saying for years to the UN that we should reschedule psychedelics," she says, referring to reports she's commissioned on global drug policies and the UN conventions that guide them. "At the moment they're in the most dangerous category of compounds. My aim was to distinguish the category of compounds like cannabis and psychedelics from other drugs," she says, so that scientists might once again revisit the work that had been interrupted. While there are several organizations around the world that fund the study of psychedelic substances, the Beckley Foundation is no doubt the greatest supporter of research on LSD.

"I personally think LSD is the most favorable [psychedelic to study], and it would be considered the most favorable had it not been under fifty years of taboo, which is why I specialize in it. That, and a commitment I made to Albert Hofmann," she says.

Feilding isn't wrong about the effects of stigma. But a scientist who has done much work for the Beckley Foundation, Robin Carhart-Harris, says he's not entirely sure LSD stands out as favorable among other compounds, particularly because of its long-lasting effects. "It's not clear that LSD has any obvious therapeutic advantages; I think I'd leave a question mark there," says Carhart-Harris, though he does acknowledge the existing body of evidence of its efficacy for alcohol dependence. When it comes to true psychedelic doses (that is, a dose that elicits a full-blown psychedelic experience), psilocybin is currently favored over LSD in clinical settings, he notes.

LSD and Microdosing

MICRODOSING INVOLVES TAKING a dose of acid (or any psychedelic) so small that the effects are imperceptible on a conscious level. (See the first case study in this chapter, with

Paul Austin, for a detailed description of how microdosing plays out in real life.) There are thousands of anecdotal reports from people around the world suggesting that microdosing with LSD or psilocybin helps with mood regulation and cognition, performance enhancement, and more. (While some studies with experimental models have tried to determine the role of the placebo effect in those who microdose, no conclusive research exists at the time of writing.) Particularly with LSD, microdosing first gained popularity among innovators and creatives in Silicon Valley, and has since been endorsed by everyone from Instagram life coaches to lawyers. On social media and forums, massive online communities of microdosers tout its benefits. Many credit their decision to experiment with microdosing to psychologist James Fadiman, whom we met several pages ago as the "father" of the phenomenon.

According to Fadiman, Albert Hofmann himself often microdosed, and believed that smaller, subperceptual doses of LSD were "under-researched." Writes Fadiman: "Had Sandoz been more interested, [Hofmann] felt that they might have had a product more useful and safer than Ritalin or its descendant Adderall."[16] Fadiman has been collecting self-study reports from individuals around the world since 2010. With LSD, his most common recommendation is to take a microdose of 10 micrograms once every four days. While all data collected is anecdotal, the list of improved health conditions that individuals have reported is not short. Fadiman has worked with a team of researchers to help turn these reports into data.

"A microdose is a very small amount of a classical psychedelic like LSD or psilocybin or mescaline," says Fadiman, speaking with me from his home in California. "And when I say very small, it's one tenth or one twentieth of what's called a recreational dose. It has no classic psychedelic effects at all. It doesn't have visions, it doesn't have profound breakthroughs of trauma and psychological issues, it doesn't have giant snakes that will eat you. It simply seems to make your mental and physical system function more effectively."

You might be asking why, if microdosing has such great potential benefits, it's not done daily. The reason is related to tolerance, notes Fadiman.

"If you take a particularly high dose of a psychedelic on Monday, and your life is transformed, and on Tuesday, you say, 'I'd like to go back there,' and you take twice as much, you don't quite go back there, but you still feel pretty good. If, on Wednesday, you do it again, nothing happens," he says. "That's what tolerance is, and the notion, by having days where you're not using a psychedelic, your system readjusts." Based on Fadiman's research, microdosing LSD is what he calls a two-day phenomenon, meaning that the positive effects of the microdose last beyond just one day. "For a number of people, the second day is even better," he says, directly quoting some of the reports he's received. The third day of the protocol, or the "second day off," gives an opportunity to return to baseline, "so they would feel the experience again on day four," or the second microdose day of the week. Many reports he received noted that after a month of microdosing, there was very little difference in effects between days one, two, and three. "They felt that their system had improved," he says.

The most common effect people experience, he observes, is more time feeling happy. Especially among people who suffer from symptoms of depression, this is huge. Fadiman makes the important distinction that unlike antidepressants, which decrease depression but also suppress emotions in general, microdosing allows people to experience improvements not only in normal depression measurements, but also in positive moods. "So, you're not only less sad," says Fadiman, "but you're more glad. The most common statement is 'I'm back.' Their normal emotional range, their full deck of cards, is available, and it's not suppressed." Fadiman says that, as with any treatment, not all people who try microdosing find it helpful, and in examining the reports he's received, he's noted that people who struggle with anxiety sometimes describe feeling increased anxiety, or becoming more aware of it.

With ongoing research and increasing commercial interest, Fadiman is hopeful that microdosing will gain ground as a useful practice, but he thinks it's unlikely microdosing will truly be taken seriously until a major pharmaceutical company "gets the message that this is the next generation [of drugs] they've been talking about."

While there are very few studies focusing on microdosing, and specifically on microdosing with LSD, one paper published in *Clinical Pharmacology & Therapeutics* in 2021 compared a placebo with doses of 5, 10, and 20 micrograms of LSD. A total of twenty-three healthy participants were used in the double-blind, placebo-controlled crossover study. At just 5 micrograms, the study authors observed an absence of relevant effects, but once doubled to 10 micrograms, participants confirmed feelings of being "under the influence" and "good drug effects," observations that are in line with previous research. A dose of 20 micrograms induced weak "but clearly significant" subjective effects when compared with smaller doses and the placebo. The authors suggest that further studies consider the effects of the 10-to-25-microgram range.[17]

Case Study
A Name Change,
a Life Change

Since her first major experience with LSD, Pantha Vohra has had many a trip, spanning the spectrum from beautiful, moving, and enlightening to dark, lonely, and frightening. One trip on the far end of this spectrum sticks out in her mind as the most defining experience of her life—one that led to a profound shift in her physical, mental, and spiritual well-being.

After a few semesters at the University of British Columbia, she decided she'd embark on her first big LSD experience while attending an outdoor music festival in Oregon. With two good friends by her side, she took a dose of liquid acid and soon began to feel her surroundings change. During the march to the concert grounds, rolling hills played tricks on her eyes, and she felt as though she'd been thrust into Wonderland. Then a fellow festivalgoer in a Cheshire Cat costume entered her line of sight, and she was convinced in that moment that she'd become Alice.

It wasn't long before Vohra became separated from her friends in the sea of people, and soon she befriended a woman who whisked her away from the concert grounds to a private tent, where she was led through a guided sound bath, a meditative experience involving singing bowls and gongs. This marked the beginning of an epic, daylong "healing journey," she says to me over FaceTime, "where every step of the trip was a different part of my life." At certain points, she felt as though all the trauma and pain she'd ever lived with was being pulled from her body and spread out into the ground.

"She told me, 'Your spirit is a panther, but you are wounded—a big, wounded, solitary animal—and that's why you feel so much pain,' " Vohra recalls. " 'Your power is that you can feel everybody's emotions, but it is also your weakness.' " After the twelve-hour experience, Vohra awoke from a slumber to realize that the woman she'd met was nowhere to be found. For the rest of the festival, their paths would not cross.

Feeling empowered by the mystical experience that expanded her mind and changed her perspective, Vohra came to feel dissociated from her given name, and decided to lean into the message she'd received.

"This trip," she says, "was the reason why I changed my name." Following her experience, Vohra experimented with microdosing and found that she benefited from taking small, imperceptible doses of acid, especially when it came to improving her perspective and developing a better understanding of the rigid, orthodox society she grew up in. Microdosing also helped integrate some of the lessons she'd learned on that first trip, many of them related to nature. Eventually, they inspired her to return to university to study forestry, so she could learn and eventually teach others about the ways that nature affects mental health.

"Had I not taken LSD, I would not be the person that I am today," she says. "I would not be as open-minded, as compassionate, or as spiritual."

What the Science Says About . . .

LSD AND
END-OF-LIFE ANXIETY

A DOUBLE-BLIND, RANDOMIZED, active placebo–controlled study published in 2015 examined the efficacy and safety of LSD in conjunction with psychotherapy for end-of-life anxiety, with promising results.[18] Over the course of three months, participants suffering from life-threatening diseases underwent between six and eight LSD-assisted psychotherapy sessions, receiving either 200 micrograms or 20 micrograms (the active placebo) during two assisted sessions. Interviews with those who received the higher dose found that all said they benefited from LSD-assisted psychotherapy, with 77.8 percent reporting sustained reductions in their anxiety, and about the same number reporting a reduced fear of death. Most participants reported improved quality of life, and experienced personality changes such as increased openness, deepened awareness, and greater patience.

Not a single patient reported lasting negative effects from the LSD experiences. It was common among participants to feel greater access to their own emotions, leading to a cathartic release. "It encouraged me to let the feelings flow... to free myself from my fears, to look at my grief," said one participant in an interview about her sessions. "It was necessary. It was relieving. Afterward I was able to laugh about it. It is a fluctuating world of emotions you have to pass during these eight hours." Others said they were able to grapple with the idea of death, viewing it through a new lens and coming to new conclusions about its relationship to life. "Dying is as usual or unusual as life itself. You cannot separate it," said another. "I simply have to familiarize myself with the idea and the process. And for that an LSD session is of priceless worth."

LSD AND DEPRESSION
AND ANXIETY

A 2019 REVIEW of classical psychedelics for depression and anxiety looks at how different psychedelics affected depression and anxiety levels in patients with either one or both conditions.

It discusses the previously mentioned study on end-of-life anxiety, noting that LSD produced immediate and significant antidepressant and anxiolytic effects, which lasted for months after the experience. You may be thinking, "Isn't LSD known to cause fits of anxiety? What about all these horror stories?" This study notes that "compared to psilocybin, LSD is thought to be more emotionally intense, with higher risk of inducing paranoia. Although this can result in severe anxiety and panic attacks at high doses, administration in the medical setting with appropriate psychological support normally safeguards against this."[19] (This point is repeated over and over in studies on LSD.)

One 1966 study that discusses the psychiatric use of LSD reported that depression "due to situational factors [is] favorably influenced... Patients with anxiety or problems of passivity or aggressivity are amenable to treatment."[20] Sidney Cohen, the same researcher who warned of LSD's potential danger, is referenced in this study as suggesting that psychopathic character disorders can be improved with LSD treatment. Other trials from the same era consider LSD as a treatment for what were referred to as "neurotic" symptoms, including anxiety, depression, and psychosomatic diseases, and found that participants reported improved symptoms six months and one year following their initial treatment.[21]

LSD'S VARYING EFFECTS

A STUDY PUBLISHED in *Neuropsychopharmacology* in 2021 addresses LSD's ability to provide different effects at different doses. It was the first study to compare the effects of 100 micrograms and 200 micrograms, both of which are considered true psychedelic doses. A total of sixteen healthy subjects took part in the double-blind, randomized, placebo-controlled, crossover study, each of them receiving six sessions: one with a placebo, another with LSD and 40 milligrams of the drug ketanserin, an antagonist or blocker of the 5-HT2A receptor, and a session each with 25, 50, 100, and 200 micrograms of LSD.

Results showed that participants experienced effects at the 25-microgram dose, and that, as expected, as the dose increased, so too did the level of effect. The study authors noted a "ceiling effect" of positive subjective effects at the 100-microgram dose, as there was no difference in positive effects between the 100 and 200 microgram doses. Interestingly, while the 200-microgram dose induced significant anxiety, it also produced signifi- cantly greater ego dissolution than the 100-microgram dose. When ketanserin was administered one hour before the 200-microgram dose, effects of LSD were significantly reduced, confirming the role of the 5-HT2A receptor, which mediates the psychedelic effects of classic psychedelics including LSD, psilocybin, DMT, and mescaline.

At the smaller dose of 50 micrograms, substantial positive mood effects were noted, with no anxiety, but also "very small and nonsignificant anxious ego dissolution." The authors of this study suggest, based on their data and the data in previ- ous research, that a dose of 100 micrograms would likely be selected for use in trials related to depression and anxiety, while the 50-microgram dose "would likely be a good starting dose to be used in patients with no previous experience with psy- chedelics," or in those who are more sensitive to the effects of psychedelic drugs. At 25 micrograms, effects were distinguish- able from placebo and "clearly acutely psychoactive in the majority of subjects," but were considerably more subtle than at 50 and 100 micrograms.[22]

Peter Van der Heyden, who has worked in the lab with LSD for decades, believes there's no such thing as a standard dose of acid.

"Unlike other substances, it has this range of dosage, going from mere micrograms up to what are potential heroic doses, well over a milligram," he tells me in an interview, describing the differences between a microdose and a "museum" dose, the name some psychedelic users have given to the dose range that is the next step up from imperceptible while avoiding a full-blown trip.

"When you start getting above 100 micrograms, it has yet a different effect. From there, as the dose increases, we see psychedelic effects involving ego loss, mystical-type experiences, and so on." Even at doses of 50 milligrams—"an unimaginable dose," but it's been done by folks who have mistaken powdered LSD for cocaine[23]—people have survived.

"To have specific types of activities across the kind of dosage range, which is orders of magnitude from one dose to another, with measurable and distinct effects at each dosage? That's astounding."

LSD AND
CESSATION OF ALCOHOL USE

LSD AS AN AID to reducing alcohol misuse was one of the most studied applications of the substance in the 1950s, and was combined with psychotherapy at several clinics in North America at the time. A more contemporary meta-analysis from 2012, looking at cessation and reduction in alcohol consumption after psychedelic use, found that across six randomized, controlled trials administering a single dose of LSD ranging from 3 micrograms per kilogram of body weight, to 800 micrograms, those who received LSD had greater odds of reporting improvement at follow-up sessions than those who received placebos.[24]

In a 2019 study that considered how effective psychedelics could be at assisting with alcohol cessation, scientists at Johns

Hopkins University conducted a cross-sectional, anonymous online survey looking for prospective participants who had overcome alcohol or drug addiction after a psychedelic experience.[25] Of 343 people included in the sample, 38 percent said they had used LSD. What's interesting is that while all had taken moderate-to-high doses intended for some sort of psychological or spiritual exploration, just 10 percent said they had intended to reduce or quit drinking alcohol by using a psychedelic. Just under 30 percent of total respondents said the psychedelic experience led to a change in their values or priorities, leading them to give up alcohol. Some also said the psychedelic experience made it easier to believe that the long-term benefits of not drinking would outweigh immediate desires, while others said it helped them believe in their own ability to stop.

Most respondents (89 percent) said they had no persisting negative feelings after their psychedelic experience. While symptoms of alcohol withdrawal were experienced by between 52 and 58 percent of the group, many said that their symptoms were less severe than before they had taken the psychedelic. Based on their answers, 83 percent of respondents no longer met the criteria for alcohol use disorder at the end of the study.

LSD AND
PAIN PERCEPTION

ALTHOUGH THE SUBJECT didn't receive much attention during the first wave of psychedelic research, some studies have shown that acid can relieve pain in terminally ill patients. A small, randomized, double-blind, placebo-controlled study published in 2021 followed up on this body of work, revealing what it describes as "the minimal dose at which analgesic activity of LSD is effective." Over the period of four days, a group of twenty-four healthy volunteers received doses of 5, 10, and 20 micrograms of LSD—doses that intentionally would not cause any mind-altering effects—as well as a placebo. Results showed that a dose of 20 micrograms significantly reduced pain perception compared with placebo, while doses at smaller increments did not. At the larger dose, pain tolerance was increased by about 20 percent. The effects of the relatively small dose on pain tolerance were equally strong when measured at ninety minutes and five hours after administration. While the study was able to show that relatively small doses of LSD could be useful in pain management, scientists are still not sure how the compound influences pain perception, although the paper's authors suggest it may have to do with the way LSD alters neural processes. It could alternatively be related to LSD's tendency to promote self-transcendence: "in essence, no self, no pain."[26]

3. DMT and Ayahuasca

SPIRIT MOLECULE, MEDICINE OF THE AMAZON

Case Study
From a Life of Panic
to a Life of Awe

When Kay Hanen first learned about the DMT-containing psychoactive brew ayahuasca, she was at the lowest point in her life. As a teenager, she'd been diagnosed with panic disorder, dysthymia (chronic low mood), and bipolar disorder, and for over a decade since then, she'd spent every day on a series of medications that numbed her out and came with unbearable side effects.

"I went to my psychiatrist, and they offered me another medication to deal with the side effects of one of my prescriptions, and that's when I knew it was all wrong," she says. The idea of taking a medication for another medication didn't feel good to Hanen, who had been living under the haze of different drugs for years. She decided to slowly taper off her medications and search for alternative therapies, first experimenting with transcranial magnetic stimulation and considering electroconvulsive therapy.

"I was having panic attacks every day, sometimes multiple times a day, and self-injuring. I wasn't able to function at all," she says. A few weeks later, Hanen attended a local conference and met the organizer, a clinical counselor and plant medicine facilitator. She had once been in the same shoes as Hanen and jumped at the opportunity to help her navigate her pain. After a few therapy sessions, Hanen learned about ayahuasca, and decided she had nothing to lose. She had seen it portrayed on TV and knew to expect vomiting, but admits that going down an internet rabbit hole in the hope of learning more only left her more confused.

"I just decided that I was going to go into it with as much of an open mind as possible... I'd been told to trust that the medicine would give me what I needed, and that was a new idea for me, because most of my experiences in life had taught me not to trust anything," she says. Arriving at the ceremony space built in a large rec room in the facilitator's home, Hanen sat near the back of the group of twenty people and was immediately comforted by the diversity of the crowd, ranging from young to old, and from experienced to new to plant medicine. When the time came for her to drink the ayahuasca, her intention was clear.

"I knew intuitively that I needed to ask to feel the love of the universe, to feel the love that everyone else feels, so that's what I asked for." As the medicine took hold, Hanen felt more in touch with her body, a feeling that was wildly unfamiliar to her: "A lot of trauma and emotions get caught in the body, and before ayahuasca, I felt cut off, like my head was a separate entity. Just the sensation of feeling the medicine move through my body was very strange... I had this intense sense of presence that felt very purposeful."

Amid the nausea she'd anticipated and the cacophony of sounds you might expect at an ayahuasca ceremony—

singing, yelling, crying, laughing, and vomiting—Hanen felt another new sensation: a feeling of focus. As her body cycled between waves of nausea and intense feelings of relief, she had a realization that would stick with her.

"That cycling reminded me of what life is, that you have to feel the lows to feel the highs. So what was stopping me from feeling them?" she recalls asking herself. Soon, the nausea climaxed with a purge that brought more than relief; Hanen felt as though she was enveloped in warmth and light, and the love she'd asked for began to pour into her.

"I heard a message very clearly: 'You are here now, and you don't have to try anymore.' I felt in my body that the trying and the striving and the wanting for things to be different was preventing me from feeling that love in every moment. Once I felt it, it was undeniable." For the rest of the ceremony, Hanen experienced awe and intense catharsis, laughing and crying at the realization she'd come to: "If I could feel this wonderful with the medicine, then I could feel this way without it."

Today, she has a deep sense of self-acceptance. She hasn't suffered from a single panic attack since that first ceremony— now several years ago—and the thoughts of suicide that once plagued her are gone.

"It felt like I was in the ocean, like I was drowning. Maybe I'd come up for a breath every now and then, but I felt suffocated by life," she says. "Now I feel like I've got a surfboard."

How Ayahuasca and DMT Work

AYAHUASCA, A POWERFUL psychoactive brew revered by more than a hundred Indigenous groups across South America, is unique in its requirement of two plants to produce psychoactive effects: the leaves of the *Psychotria viridis* or chacruna shrub, and the stalks of the *Banisteriopsis caapi* vine, often referred to as "the ayahuasca vine." The leaves of *Psychotria viridis* contain the powerful psychedelic substance *N,N*-dimethyltryptamine, or DMT. Unfortunately, DMT is a chemical compound with relatively low bioavailability, meaning once it is consumed, it is metabolized quickly before the active chemical reaches the brain. If consumed orally, it will not lead to a psychedelic experience, because enzymes in the gut and liver called monoamine oxidases, or MAOs, work fast to break it down. This is where *Banisteriopsis caapi* comes in: this plant contains MAO inhibitors, or MAOIs, that block the enzymes and allow DMT to enter the bloodstream and make its way to the brain. These MAOIs are referred to as beta-carboline alkaloids. One alkaloid that blocks the enzymes that would otherwise break down DMT is called harmine, and it also has psychoactive properties. Recipes differ from region to region, and other plants may be included in the brew; however, these two ingredients are crucial for ayahuasca's signature four-to-six-hour journey.[1]

At the molecular level, DMT—a classic psychedelic—has a structure similar to serotonin's and an affinity for some serotonin receptors. It is an agonist of the 5-HT2A and 5-HT1A sites. Research shows that it also has an affinity for the Sigma-1 receptor (S1R), which is involved in the promotion of neural plasticity,[2] the nervous system's ability to change in response to stimuli by reorganizing its structure, functions, and connections. It has also been implicated in conditions including depression, substance use disorder, amnesia, and pain. A 2015 study of ten participants who had each regularly used ayahuasca utilized MRI scans and found that the part of the brain housing the default mode network had been affected in a way that is believed to result in reduced anxiety and apprehension, and increased introspection.[3]

Administration, Dosing,
and Effects of Ayahuasca and DMT

AYAHUASCA (WHICH CONTAINS DMT) is administered as a tea, while DMT synthesized in a lab can be administered on its own, either by smoking or via injection. Doses of ayahuasca vary depending on the potency of the brew. Generally, people who participate in ayahuasca ceremonies do not decide their own dose. Instead, a *curandero* or healer will administer an initial dose, and may later give participants an opportunity to drink another cup.

Once ayahuasca is consumed, it generally takes thirty minutes for its effects to take hold. The onset can be unpleasant, with a burning or acidic sensation in the stomach, as well as hot and cold flashes, yawning, and a feeling of pins and needles in the skin. Purging or vomiting is also common with ayahuasca. Within forty-five or sixty minutes, visualizations begin to take place, most often behind closed eyes—although some people will go through an entire ayahuasca journey without having any visualizations at all.[4] (This is not uncommon, and one should not draw the conclusion that not having visions means the drug is not working.) The ayahuasca experience peaks at around ninety minutes to two hours,[5] and ends after four to six hours. Senses are heightened, and the introspective state brought on by the brew helps the psyche make new associations, while promoting reflection on one's life, including personal issues, buried memories, and emotions.

When DMT is consumed outside of ayahuasca—that is, when it's smoked or administered via intravenous infusion—the onset of effects is extremely rapid, but these effects last for a much shorter period, no longer than thirty to forty-five minutes.[6] Average doses depend on how the drug is administered. When smoked, average recreational doses reportedly vary from 30 to 150 milligrams; when administered intravenously in study settings, doses have ranged from 0.05 to 0.4 milligrams of DMT per kilogram of body weight. The effects of DMT when smoked or injected are almost instant, taking the user to a realm far beyond this one. They include intense visual and auditory hallucinations or visualizations, euphoria, and altered states of self, space, and time. Many people describe visiting alternative realities and seeing otherworldly beings such as angels and elves. (This ability to induce spiritual or religious experiences is why DMT has earned the nickname "the spirit molecule.")

The unpleasant side effects that can come with either drinking ayahuasca or taking DMT include increased heart rate, increased blood pressure, agitation, rapid eye movements, dizziness, and nausea. In addition to vomiting or purging, it may cause diarrhea. DMT is not considered habit-forming, but it does pose other serious risks. Using DMT or ayahuasca can put some individuals, especially those who are taking antidepressants, at risk of serotonin syndrome, an overaccumulation of serotonin in the body that can lead to high blood pressure, loss of coordination, confusion, and even death. Responsible ayahuasca centers and facilities will require potential visitors to submit detailed medical histories. Question (and consider avoiding) any setting where ayahuasca is served without close consideration of medical history.

Diving Deep:
The DMT Experience

AFTER PSYCHEDELIC SCIENCE had been dead in the water for more than twenty years, psychiatrist Rick Strassman was among the first to pursue psychedelic research, particularly on the effect that the compound DMT has on humans. Strassman's work was the result of a long-standing interest in what he refers to as "the biology of the spiritual experience."

"I went to school on the West Coast in the late '60s and early '70s, and there was an influx of new technologies that could reliably cause profound altered states of consciousness. Those were meditation and psychedelic drugs," he says when he speaks to me from his home in New Mexico. "There was overlap between the descriptions of these two 'syndromes' as it were, so I began wondering if there was some biological basis for those overlaps." Strassman began by looking at the pineal gland. At the time, very little was known about this part of the brain, but Strassman had noted its long history of importance in esoteric physiologies. (Seventeenth-century philosopher René Descartes called it "the seat of the soul"; others have referred to it as "the third eye.") He started his clinical research career with an exhaustive study of the function of human melatonin, a hormone synthesized and secreted by the pineal gland that helps maintain the body's circadian rhythm. He then dived into DMT, which he believed was also produced by the gland. He applied for permission and funding to give DMT in a psychopharmacological dose-response study to measure the effects of different doses on mood, sensation, thinking, and behavior. The study began in 1990. It helped that he was working at the University of New Mexico, where the chairman of the ethics board was a strict libertarian who once told Strassman, "If it's good science, we're not playing God."

"I got a lot of support," remembers Strassman. "The DEA gave me my permit, and the FDA was actually excited that a good study was coming for the first time in twenty years." Because Strassman was the first to revisit psychedelics with a trial, there was no existing framework for performing a Schedule I drug study in humans, and while he says dealing with federal agencies was at times difficult, "it wasn't because of resistance—it was because of regulatory inertia."

The scientific community was caught completely off guard by Strassman's work: "Some of the people who'd studied psychedelics in the '60s would come up to me and say, 'It's déjà vu all over again.' People didn't want to get that close. But I never really got much pressure or publicity."

Strassman hypothesized that if giving DMT to normal volunteers produced states of consciousness resembling nondrug states—that is, if it replicated certain features of a nondrug religious experience or a near-death experience—this would be evidence for naturally occurring DMT. "In other words, in both conditions, there are elevated levels of DMT in the brain," he says. Even though his study was funded by the National Institute on Drug Abuse, his strict focus was on psychopharmacology dose-response work. The study involved nearly five dozen healthy participants, all of whom had had a prior psychedelic experience. Each participant received low, medium, and high doses administered via intravenous infusion.

"It starts within a few heartbeats," says Strassman of the intense high that is characteristic of DMT. "People described a rush, a building up of speed and internal pressure. It was kind of anxiety provoking; your heart would start to beat quite hard and fast. Accompanying the rush was a high-pitched sound. If your eyes were open, the room would start to break down visually into pixelations, overlying kaleidoscopic patterns forming in the air and on surfaces." (This proved to be distract-ing, so within a month of beginning the study, participants were given eyeshades.) The rush climaxed after forty-five sec-onds or a minute, and then participants described feeling as though they had been catapulted out of their bodies, losing complete awareness of their physical form. Each participant had their blood pressure taken at two minutes and five minutes into the dose. No one was aware of the check at two minutes, and only a few participants were cognizant of the check at five minutes.

"You lose complete awareness of your body, and you're transported into this world of light—rapidly moving, incredi-bly saturated. There's content, and there is interaction. There isn't just 'a white light,' and you're not dissolved into it. You're still there; your personality, your will, your mind is completely there, and you're observing, interacting, and communicating. There is an intelligence in that space, and sometimes these intelligences would coalesce into a discernible being: a cactus, a human, robots. These beings would possess intelligence and power, and they were aware of you."

Strassman says that although a few participants said they felt panicked, most described the experience as intense but generally positive. (Note that this study was conducted with healthy volunteers, and not in the interest of psychotherapy—so, unlike some of the studies that are being conducted today, "there were no bells and whistles, no incense, no comfy room," as Strassman points out.) Between two and five minutes, par-ticipants "peaked," and then experienced a come-down around the ten-minute mark. Thirty minutes after the DMT had been administered, most participants were able to converse nor-mally—though Strassman says many were astonished to learn how little time had passed during their experience.

"For some, it was a lifetime of experience—like a thousand years—but for everybody, it seemed a lot longer than it was." Another commonality was the conviction that participants had about their experiences: "There was a feeling of certainty that what they were witnessing was more real than real . . . more solid, more convincing, more undeniable, than everyday reality." Another conclusion of the study was that, unlike other psychedelics, "DMT was not inherently anything. It wasn't inherently spiritual, it wasn't therapeutic—it just catapulted people into this state."

Strassman stresses that DMT and the psychedelic experience in general is less "mind-expanding" than it is "mind-manifesting"—that is, "it isn't good or bad, it just amplifies or clarifies the things that are already in your mind." ("Expanding," he says later on in our conversation, "depends on the set and setting." If the deck isn't stacked in favor of a positive experience, Strassman says, using DMT can have a constricting rather than an expanding effect on the mind, countering the notion that all psychedelic trips result in feelings of peace and love.)

"It could be that the psychedelic just makes whatever is in your mind already more true, more convincing. If you're a peaceful person and you take DMT, you'll be even more convinced how important it is to be peaceful . . . it doesn't put anything into your mind that isn't already there."

While Strassman was interested in further exploring the spiritual effects of DMT, it was the early '90s, and he was a one-man operation without access to the team of psychologists he'd need to do so. The good news is his research has paved the way for today's scientists to take a closer look at DMT dosing. While the scope of Strassman's work did not include examining its effects on neurogenesis, a 2020 study showed that the drug can trigger the growth of new brain cells in mice.[7]

"There are increasing amounts of data indicating the neuro-genesis effects of psychedelics, including DMT." Strassman further explains: "[They] increase complexity of connections among nerve cells and stimulate the growth of new nerve cells." He predicts that future research will examine both psychedelic and subperceptual doses of the drug, as well as infusions that last longer than the average DMT trip. Because the drug is so short-acting, it doesn't allow for much therapeutic work to be done (though Strassman doesn't discount anecdotes he's heard from people with substance use issues who smoked DMT and had experiences so profound that they stopped using drugs.) He says in order to better characterize the drug's effects, future studies could use continuous infusions of DMT for sessions that are closer in length to an ayahuasca experience (around six hours). More time in the DMT state, he says, may allow greater benefit to the recipient.

A Closer Look:
The Ayahuasca Experience

WHILE AYAHUASCA CONTAINS the active compound DMT, experiences with either are not interchangeable. "Ayahuasca is a combinatory plant psychedelic that has a long history of use for healing and divination in the Amazon, and it's the only psychedelic known to require two plants," says ethnobotanist Chris Kilham when we talk on the phone. Kilham is the author of *The Ayahuasca Test Pilots Handbook*, as well as several other books about medicinal plants. Since his first experience with ayahuasca, in which he was relieved of lifelong grief over his mother's death, Kilham has advocated for sustainable plant medicine harvesting practices, and has worked closely with local communities to conduct field studies in the Peruvian

Amazon. Since 1994, he has drunk ayahuasca with more than sixty shamans. Together with his wife, Zoe Helene, founder of psychedelic feminist collective Cosmic Sister, Kilham travels to the Amazon regularly as part of a collaborative project called Ayahuasca Test Pilots. For Kilham, journeying with ayahuasca is a sacred ceremonial experience, and one that should not be taken lightly.

"Ayahuasca peels back the layers of who you are," he says. "It not only shows you difficult things about yourself, or things that need to be resolved or healed; it shows you the really wonderful things about yourself. The truth-telling that you get with ayahuasca, if you choose to carry it forward and do something about it, is powerfully transformative. In a great many ways, it's been informative and transformative for me."

One misconception Kilham often hears from the ayahuasca-curious is over what they might "see": "I've heard many people express concern that they might not have visions, and that's kind of a funny worry. You don't have to have visions to heal; you don't have to have visions to get good guidance on ways to improve your life and move forward." Kilham's deep relationship with ayahuasca informs his understanding of how the potent psychedelic brew works, and he is a strong believer in the idea that there is much more going on than a chemical reaction.

"There are a lot of people who think of ayahuasca as a chemical only, and this is where we really have diverging ways of thinking with regard to plants: some people who are theoretical experts in this field insist that it's purely a matter of harmala alkaloids and DMT getting together and reacting in your body. I don't buy that for a second," says the ethnobotanist. "Through the guidance and thoughtfulness of really talented shamans, I do accept there is a plant spirit, and I think there is a lack of understanding of how extraordinarily valuable that is. You can't put ayahuasca in a box."

Helene, a respected and widely recognized advocate for plant medicines and their keepers, has also had several experiences with ayahuasca, and says that while it's understandable people might have some fear of the nausea and purging from drinking it, these things are all part of the healing process.

"It's this cultural idea of not wanting to drink something 'nasty' and puke into a bucket, but that's part of the tradition of the medicine," she says. "I have had so many experiences personally where I puked up some things that I needed to leave behind in that bucket, things that had to leave my psyche so I could heal them." The lack of purging and the shorter duration associated with DMT might appeal to some people, Helene notes, but she considers DMT just one part of something that is much better experienced holistically.

"You know the phrase 'An apple a day keeps the doctor away'? It's the whole apple. It's not just the skin, or just the tasty part— it's all of the above," she says. "It's the set and setting. It's the agreement you make with yourself to suspend disbelief, and with others who are participating. It's releasing judgment, it's your intention, and it's the *dieta* [diet] you do to prepare," she adds, emphasizing that the latter—a pre-ceremony ritual involving a vegetarian diet with no sugar, spices, oils, alcohol, fermented foods, or sex—is about preparing not just the body but the psyche. It's important, she says, to watch what you put into your mind before you consume ayahuasca. "You're not necessarily going to get all of that with DMT. I'm not saying that it's bad; it's just completely different. Plus, the longer ride with ayahuasca gives you much more time to investigate."

Both Kilham and Helene stress that those who feel called to drink ayahuasca should do ample research and weigh options thoughtfully before deciding on a preferred setting. The popularization of the sacred brew since the 1990s has made Iquitos, Peru, the "capital of ayahuasca" and a hub of retreat centers, a destination that draws as many ill-intentioned visitors and shamans as it does those who are genuinely seeking and guiding healing. Without the right support, an experience with ayahuasca can lead to more internal disharmony. A trip to the Amazon might seem like the best option for some, but for others, the stress of traveling to another country and being in the presence of strangers may not make for the best experience. Another reason one might prefer to stay local is that it can be easier to verify a shaman's history through word of mouth and the experiences of friends than to do so over the internet. The popularization of ayahuasca has led to underground ceremonies in every major city from Los Angeles to Lima, so if staying local is more within your comfort zone, there are options—but tapping into these communities can take some networking.

Making sure you're in trustworthy hands is important, because at times the feeling of being on ayahuasca—or any psychedelic—can become physically incapacitating. Sexual abuse has been reported in a small percentage of cases both in and outside the Amazon, in which individuals have been coerced into removing their clothes or worse.[8] (Such demands are in no way customary of the ayahuasca ritual, but as these reports have noted, people who are abused in these situations often fear that they won't be believed if they speak up.) Abuse in therapeutic settings is not limited to ayahuasca rituals or even drug-assisted psychotherapy, but psychedelics can widen the power imbalance between a therapist/practitioner and the person under their influence. (This is in part why, in most clinical research and at many treatment centers where psychedelics are offered, two therapists are assigned to every patient.)[9] The need for safeguards against abuse and practices that reduce harm has never been greater, and this is being increasingly recognized throughout the psychedelic community. In an effort to help prevent abuses, practitioners are creating ethics councils and formalized reporting processes so that victims of abuse feel safe to come forward.[10] Whether pursuing psychedelics in a regulated or unregulated setting, don't be afraid to ask questions. Any reluctance to answering questions about safety or personal space should be a red flag.

So what exactly does one investigate during a deep journey with ayahuasca? Helene has recently been exploring what she calls "ancestor medicine," an unlearning and relearning of who she is through her ancestral lineage—and it's something she's encouraging other people who use psychedelics to do.

"I see so many others, not just me, really suffering from this sense of 'Who the fuck am I?' " she says. You might be wondering what the value is in revisiting the history of your lineage, especially if it's one full of trauma, while on a psychedelic journey, but Helene says this sort of exploration can provide an opportunity to better understand not only who we are, but *why* we are. As she writes on the Cosmic Sister website: "Exploring ancestry with the help of sacred plant allies can be empowering in surprising ways. Delving deeply into our individual and collective past can help inform choices we make in the present." For Helene, whose mother is Greek and father is Jewish and Scottish, working with psychedelics in this way has been both "profoundly healing and profoundly difficult," and highly relevant to her work in running an organization that stands on pillars of antiracism, feminism, and environmentalism: "It's relevant to everyone. If you're not indigenous to where you are living, you're either an immigrant or a refugee." Ancestor medicine, she says, need not only be considered within a psychedelic journey. It can be as simple as creating the intention to connect with your lineage while in a meditation, and as complicated as having your DNA tested and planning a real-life trip to places where your ancestors lived. The idea is that the work itself is the medicine. Helene's current exploration of her ancestry is worth bringing up, because as more and more people become interested in working with psychedelic plant medicines that have long-standing traditions outside of their own cultures and homelands, the issue of cultural appropriation arises again and again, especially in psychedelic communities in North America. It's important to respect the fact that some traditions and rituals are sacred, and only accessible to those within certain cultures. Getting in touch with one's own lineage, either within a psychedelic experience or by some other means, helps answer the daunting question "Who am I?" while (hopefully) increasing awareness of appropriation, belonging, and the rights of Indigenous peoples with respect to their traditions and rituals.

Ayahuasca and DMT: Early Use

LIKE OTHER PLANT and fungus medicines mentioned in this book, ayahuasca—also referred to as yagé, caapi, yajé, and aya—has likely been used for thousands of years by Indigenous groups and Mestizo cultures, particularly those in the northwestern region of the Amazon basin. These groups include the Shipibo, the Yaminawá, the Huni Kuin, the Tsáchila, the Chachi, the Emberá, the Chocó, and the Yora, among over a hundred others.[11] The name *ayahuasca* comes from the Quechuan words *aya*, meaning "spirit," "soul," or "ancestor," and *huasca*, meaning "vine," translating to "vine of the soul."[12]

In the late 2000s, archaeologists excavated an ancient rock shelter in the Lípez highlands of Bolivia, where they found what would eventually be determined as evidence of ayahuasca's earliest use among humans. The shelter contained what appeared to be a shaman's ritual bundle, bearing residue of several psychoactive chemicals, including DMT and harmine. These residues were analyzed and radiocarbon-dated to 1000 CE. Prior to this discovery, harmine had been found in the hair of mummies in the Azapa Valley of northern Chile, and dated to between 400 and 900 CE. Scientists believe that this indicates these people consumed the *Banisteriopsis caapi* vine, but can't confirm whether they combined it with leaves of the chacruna shrub. Some scientists believe that the cultural practice of combining the two substances is a more recent phenomenon.[13] (It's an incredible wonder that the recipe was ever discovered, as there are more than 80,000 plant species in the Amazon.)

The Indigenous communities that use ayahuasca should in no way be considered as a single, undifferentiated group. In the Amazon basin, the shaman-led rituals accompanying the consumption of ayahuasca vary widely, and while there are similarities, there is no "true" or "authentic" ayahuasca ritual.[14] For the cultural groups that use it, ayahuasca is an integral part of their worldview, and is in many instances woven into creation stories. In the same way that the Mazatec view psilocybin mushrooms, they see ayahuasca as a plant teacher.

Documenting Ayahuasca

THE EARLIEST MENTION of ayahuasca outside the Amazon occurred in the mid-1600s, when Jesuit priests and missionaries made note of the use of ayahuasca in ritualistic ceremony. This first report, which referred to the Indigenous peoples who used ayahuasca as "sorcerers," was written in Latin by historian José Chantre y Herrera and sent to Rome.[15] The priest Pablo Maroni wrote a second report in 1737, describing ayahuasca as "an intoxicating potion ingested for divinatory and other purposes ... which deprives one of his senses, and, at times, of his life." In 1755, Franz Xavier Veigl, also a Jesuit, wrote about the psychoactive brew after encountering its use in the Amazon, describing it as "a bitter reed" which "serves for mystification and bewitchment."[16]

It was almost a century before ayahuasca was written about again. In the 1850s, Ecuadorian-born Manuel Villavicencio described his personal experience with ayahuasca, and in 1873, Richard Spruce, a botanist from England who had witnessed an ayahuasca ceremony in 1852, was the first to catalogue the plant taxonomically.

Of his experience with ayahuasca, Villavicencio wrote, "It is a vine which the [Indigenous people] use to guess, predict, and answer correctly the difficult questions ... after the last dream gathers up the memories that were in the visions, it shows you the decision you should make ... To the [person] who drinks [ayahuasca], should be given the answers ... the rarest of phenomena."[17] Spruce, a meticulous botanist who consumed ayahuasca on several occasions and even sent samples of *Banisteriopsis caapi* to England for assessment, hailed it as a plant with unique, though unknown, medical benefits: "This is all I have seen and learnt of ayahuasca. I regret being unable to tell what is the peculiar narcotic principle that produces such extraordinary effects." Unfortunately, his shipment was seized and grew moldy before reaching England for assessment, and his reports of the "vine of the soul" were not disseminated among other botanists as he'd hoped.

Still, researchers neglected ayahuasca until 1957. American biologist Richard Evans Schultes (considered the father of ethnobotany, the study of people's relationships to and traditional knowledge of plants) was the first to author an academic article on ayahuasca.[18] He hypothesized that beta-carboline alkaloids in the vine like harmine and harmaline were responsible for making the DMT active. Ten years later, at a National Institutes of Health symposium on the medical potential of psychedelic compounds, a panel discussion of experts focused on the brew from the Amazon.[19] Finally, in his 1992 book *Food of the Gods*, Terence McKenna popularized the idea (confirmed in self-experiments) that beta-carbolines "are important to visionary shamanism because they can inhibit the enzyme systems in the body that would otherwise depotentiate hallucinogens of the DMT type . . . [They] can be used in conjunction with DMT to prolong and intensify visual hallucinations. This combination is the basis of the hallucinogenic brew ayahuasca."[20]

While there is certainly more scientific interest in ayahuasca today than there was during the first wave of psychedelic study, ayahuasca has always maintained a sense of mystery in academic circles, and for good reason: as those who have drunk it will tell you, ayahuasca is a sentient being whose power and cultural importance cannot be limited to the pages of an academic paper. To call it an enigma would not be inaccurate, but that has not stopped scientists from trying to gain a better understanding of its use and components.

Ayahuasca's Appropriation: What Science Must Learn From Tradition

BIA CAIUBY LABATE is a queer Brazilian anthropologist and the founder of the Chacruna Institute, an organization that aims to educate the public about psychedelic plant medicines like ayahuasca while presenting academic knowledge on their cultural uses in a more accessible way, an effort she undertook when she became weary of the barriers in academia.

"We are very focused on the cultural sphere and creating legitimacy around these plants," she says. Labate's work focuses primarily on creating bridges between the world of Indigenous sacred-plant use, ceremony, ritual, religion, and tradition, and the emerging field of psychedelic science and psychedelic-assisted therapy, while platforming Indigenous peoples, people of color, and others who are generally not at the forefront of the mainstream psychedelic discourse.

"We're trying to rewrite the narrative that the psychedelic field tells about itself, to itself," she says. Rather than being messianic about psychedelics and claiming that they are a salvation for society, Chacruna defends the rights of those who wish to use psychedelics—but she qualifies this with an important point. "At Chacruna, what we like to say is, it's not just about our rights, it's about our obligations, because with rights come responsibilities."

In the face of growing interest from scientists and medical researchers, she suggests that science is just one mode of understanding: "Biomedical knowledge is not the only or ultimate measure of reality. It's really important to support scientific research, but it's also important to understand other disciplines. Traditional populations have empirical, firsthand knowledge of these experiences that in many cases trump a lot of the epidemiological evidence," she says. "Some of these substances are much older than the scheduling system and prohibition itself, so I think we have to advocate for an expansion [of psychedelics] that is balanced, inclusive, and responsible, while also cultivating compassion and kindness."

This, she notes, starts with involving the traditional keepers of medicines like ayahuasca in the policy discussions on their regulation, and recognizing the rights of the plants and the land on which they grow. It also involves reciprocity, and a louder and more pronounced recognition of what is owed to the Indigenous cultures that have suffered at the hands of greedy colonialists who time and time again have appropriated their cultural practices.

"Anybody and everybody in the psychedelic movement has some kind of debt to Indigenous people. We are all heirs of this tradition and this knowledge, because these Indigenous groups were the first to find these substances, to study them and bring them to our attention," she says. "So, there is a continuity between the shamanic uses, the underground therapeutic uses, and the above-ground clinical trials."

One lesson that Labate believes those who decide to take psychedelic plant medicines can learn from Indigenous peoples is a more sophisticated notion of healing.

"From an Indigenous perspective, healing is a more comprehensive affair. It involves relationship with the individual, but it also involves other individuals, the family, the community, and also with the nonhuman, with the land, with the cosmos." This more holistic approach ought to be incorporated into clinical practices with psychedelic substances, she says. Labate echoes Zoe Helene's message about ancestry, too: "Another thing that we can learn, is to look at our lineage, our ancestry. There's an importance in understanding these things, but it frequently gets lost in Western healing. Looking legitimately at our own culture and trying to reconcile our relationships as communities with Native people through decolonization is part of the mission of honoring these traditions."

Case Study
Why the Right
Support Is Critical

Today, Salimeh Tabrizi knows intrinsically that ayahuasca is not just a plant medicine teacher but a close ally that has helped her move through the intensity of life with grace, providing her with a completely "new paradigm" in healing. The clinical counselor left a company therapy practice to open her own and become "PR for the plants," making it her life's mission to advocate for them after her first journey with ayahuasca. She offers counseling as well as plant medicine preparation and integration sessions for clients seeking guidance. Looking back on her first experience several years ago, she admits that although it has helped her immensely, not having the right support around her journey with ayahuasca made the road to healing far more challenging than it needed to be.

Before she was introduced to ayahausca, Tabrizi was a happy-go-lucky woman with everything going for her, but inside she carried anxiety and repressed trauma, including childhood sexual abuse and immense resentment toward her father. She ventured to Peru on her own, in search of ayahuasca in the hope that it would help her peel back the layers of her anxiety.

"In that ceremony, I was able to hug my father for the first time after many, many years," she says from Costa Rica when we connect for an interview on Zoom. And though she admits it sounds odd, ayahuasca showed her what it was like "to be able to put my head in my own lap," a visualization that provided her with a sense of being held and supported by her higher self. But the ceremony stirred something up in Tabrizi that was not quelled by the journey's end: the repressed trauma of being hypnotized and sexually abused by a family member became crystal clear in her mind, and left her with deep feelings of rage, violation, uncertainty, and lack of trust.

"Caged animals, when the door is opened for them, have a hard time," she says. "Ayahuasca broke my mind, and although it prepared me for the light that was about to come into my life, I went into psychosis for six months." For weeks after the ceremony, Tabrizi received guidance from a therapist, but when that time came to an end, integrating what she'd learned was a painful and at times terrifying process.

"I was not really capable of making food or leaving the house. But by going through that, I now understand that it doesn't have to be like that. People don't need to go through these massive points of struggle just to heal," she says. Tabrizi has taken these lessons to heart in her work as a plant medicine integration coach and counselor, and recognizes that another crucial ingredient to any plant medicine experience, especially one with ayahuasca, is community.

"I really learned the importance of holding people for a much longer amount of time. After two days of ceremony, then what?... It was a complete rebuilding of myself and who I am, really emptying out all the traumas and fears and beliefs, so that more light could come in, and bring me to a different place." Since then, Tabrizi credits ayahuasca with helping her come into a new career, a new way of being with community, and a deeper union with her partner. She continues to follow the guidance of ayahuasca, which she refers to lovingly as her grandmother.

"Now, I understand," she says. "She knows that we can only survive through community."

What the Science Says About...

AYAHUASCA AND
DEPRESSION

IN A DOUBLE-BLIND, randomized, placebo-controlled trial conducted in Brazil, ayahuasca was given to twenty-nine participants with treatment-resistant depression between the ages of eighteen and sixty, none of whom had taken ayahuasca before. One group received a placebo—a beverage made to look and taste like ayahuasca, but containing none of the active ingredient—and another received ayahuasca supplied by a local church, all from the same batch so that dosing was consistent. Patients were weaned off SSRIs for the trial to prevent severe adverse reactions, such as serotonin syndrome.[21] Ayahuasca was administered not in a ceremonial setting but in a living-room-like environment with a bed, recliner, low lighting, and a music system.

The severity of the participants' depression was assessed before the trial and then one, two, and seven days after their session. Before the session, all patients met the criteria for moderate-to-severe depression. The researchers found that the group that was given ayahuasca experienced rapid anti-depressant effects after a single dosing session. While depression severity was alleviated in both groups, the improvements were much greater among the ayahuasca group. Both saw high response rates when assessed on day one and two but were significantly higher for the ayahuasca group on day seven. (By day seven, some symptoms of depression had returned to those in the placebo group.) All participants said they felt safe, but some noted that the ayahuasca experience was "not necessarily pleasant," and reported nausea, vomiting, and psychological distress.

(Interestingly, the substance used as placebo induced nausea and anxiety in participants as well, with a third of the patients in the group misidentifying it as ayahuasca.) While this study only monitored patients for one week following their experience, its authors indicate that even by day seven, the rate of remission among participants who received ayahuasca "showed a trend toward significance."[22] In a previous report by many of the same researchers, depression scores were taken at one, seven, and twenty-one days following an ayahuasca session. They noted reductions of symptoms of up to 82 percent.[23]

AYAHUASCA AND SUBSTANCE USE

AN OBSERVATIONAL STUDY conducted in Canada in 2013 considered how ayahuasca-assisted therapy might impact individuals suffering from substance use issues. Twelve participants living in a rural First Nations community received four days of group counseling and participated in two ayahuasca ceremonies as part of a retreat program called "Working With Addiction and Stress." Assessments were made before and six months after the experience, with researchers hypothesizing that participants would experience improvements in mindfulness, emotional regulation, personal empowerment, hopefulness, and quality of life, as well as a reduction in problematic substance use. Unlike the Brazilian study above, ayahuasca was administered in its traditional ceremonial setting, with participants following a strict diet during the four-day retreat.

Following the retreat, participants experienced statistically significant improvements in measures like mindfulness, empowerment, and hopefulness. The researchers noted reductions in the use of tobacco, alcohol, and cocaine, as well as a statistically significant reduction in problematic cocaine use. Participants also reported improved connection with themselves and with others.

"I realize that I deserve a better life and I love myself," said one participant in a follow-up interview. "I have more respect for myself. And the honesty that, just being honest with myself and others, had a major impact... [Ayahuasca] really opened my eyes. It was like I was shut down [before drinking ayahuasca]. My mind and my eyes were shut down to everything. After the retreat I felt like a brick was lifted off of my shoulders and I was just feeling free."

Another participant experienced profound changes in her relationships: "Before the ceremony I was struggling with my addiction, crack cocaine, for many years. And when I went to this retreat, it more or less helped me release the hurt and pain that I was carrying around and trying to bury that hurt and pain with drugs and alcohol. Ever since this retreat I've been clean and sober. So, it had a major impact on my life in a positive way... My family is back in my life. My daughter is back at home. And we are getting closer and closer every day as time goes on."

Another common effect of the experience was feeling a reconnection with nature: "I got my spirit back, for one," said a participant. "Nature, like it's saying, 'Wake up and smell the coffee.' Like it's so beautiful outside, and where was all that all this time? You know, I was just living [with] a black cloud over me. And the black cloud's been removed basically. Because life is a lot nicer than it ever was. You know? I go spirit bathing every morning."[24]

Another observational study, this one published in 2018, sought to assess the impact of the ceremonial use of ayahuasca on members of the União do Vegetal, or UDV, a religious society in Brazil that integrates the use of ayahuasca. This study included a much larger sample—1,947 members of the church, to be exact—and compared levels of alcohol and tobacco use with a national sample of nonmembers. The data indicated that lifetime use of alcohol and tobacco was higher among UDV members than it was in control groups for the age ranges of twenty-five to thirty-four years and over thirty-four years, but not for those aged eighteen to twenty-four. However, UDV members showed a significantly lower prevalence of disordered or problematic use of alcohol and tobacco, with even less use among those who had been members of the UDV for three years or more. The authors note that this is in line with previous data that suggests that people who use ayahuasca have lower rates of current problematic drug and alcohol use, but greater lifetime exposure to drugs. While the mechanics of the relationship between ayahuasca and substance use is not fully understood, researchers agree that ayahuasca "can modulate dependence in ways that reduce drug use and abuse patterns."[25]

AYAHUASCA AND
OUR DNA

AN EARLY-STAGE STUDY conducted by a group of researchers at King's College London and the University of Exeter asked a question that no researcher had broached in a publication before: what effect, if any, does ayahuasca have on how our genes (that is, our human DNA) are expressed? Working in collaboration with the Ayahuasca Foundation in Iquitos, Peru, an organization that works alongside the local Mishana community and was built with research in mind, researchers asked people who were already attending the foundation for a retreat if they were willing to complete surveys about their experiences. They also asked these people to submit saliva samples before and after their journey with ayahuasca.

Inventory surveys were taken before their retreats and follow-up surveys were completed six months later, measuring depression, anxiety, self-compassion, mindfulness, general well-being, and the perception of traumatic memories. The follow-ups showed that depression and anxiety had decreased, and that self-compassion, mindfulness, and general well-being had increased. Participants were likewise able to perceive memories in a more positive light.

"We also found that the greater degree their mystical experience, the greater their decrease in depression, which was in line with other psychedelic research," study author Dr. Simon Ruffell tells me when I interview him. But what was most fascinating about this study was the correlation between decreases in depression and the "statistically significant" change in SIGMAR1 gene activity they experienced post-retreat. SIGMAR1, or the sigma non-opioid intracellular receptor 1 gene, is believed to be linked to the storing of traumatic memories.[26] The authors noted that after the retreat, participants with higher scores in measures of childhood trauma had increased SIGMAR1 gene activity. Because of the small sample size, Ruffell says it's too early to draw conclusions, "but what it does suggest is that ayahuasca may well be having some kind of effect on the genetic level."

4. Mescaline and Sacred Cacti

DESERT MEDICINE FOR THE SOUL

Case Study
Advice From a Former
Sergeant at Arms

Mary Porter is the cofounder of the Looking Glass Peyote Church and a descendent of the Yakama, Wasco, and Nez Perce peoples. She lives on Klamath Modoc land in Sprague River, Oregon. Porter founded the church with her husband to provide a place for the use of peyote that relies on precontact rituals (ones that don't include elements of Christianity), based on teachings she received during the Sun Dance, a plains Indigenous cultural ceremony of renewal and sacrifice involving fasting and the endurance of pain. She was called to peyote while living a life vastly different from the one she lives today, and says it has changed her life immensely.

"Before I took the sacrament, I was a gun-toting Harley rider, and I rode with combat veterans. I was the sergeant at arms [of a motorcycle club], and a very violent, very cold person," she says. "I was called to the medicine, and since that day, my whole life has been dedicated to giving the sacrament its due, as a human being on this earth to help other human beings."

For Porter, taking peyote is akin to making a treaty, a pact, or an agreement with natural law that begins the moment the sacrament is ingested. It is not *at all* a responsibility that should be taken lightly: "You are giving your days after this to the sacrament. When you take the sacrament, you are taking the life of a sacred being. You're killing it, ingesting it, and you're becoming its afterlife. You are escorting the sacred being into your life."

Porter says that she doesn't see peyote "as something to heal you or fix you," but as something that allows you to be of service to others and the earth. This pact goes far beyond the narrative peddled by science that taking an entheogenic substance is all about human improvement.

"What I've been taught is that this is a catalyst for your spiritual evolution, almost like [what] happened when your spiritual life began in your mother's womb," she says. It's why anyone looking to take the sacrament with Porter at Looking Glass is required to fill out a questionnaire to give her an idea of where they are in their spiritual journey.

"It takes 125 years to grow this natural plant, and so there is not enough for everybody. I reserve it for those who have reached a point in their spiritual maturity where they are ready to say, 'I'm going to live my life so that this sacrament can do its job as a human being on this planet to help others.' If you're not ready to do that, you're not ready to do this." For those who *are* ready, using the sacrament can free them from the limitations and ideals forced upon them by their surroundings.

"Society projects reality upon us. That's another thing that the sacrament really peels away. Then you're allowed to have your energy that nature has prescribed for you ... Peyote is reserved strictly for people who are ready with their hands clean, their heart clear, and their mind free of the projections of this world."

More than anything, Porter stresses that those who feel compelled to use not only peyote, but any psychedelic, should be honest with themselves about why they are drawn to them. "Not everybody can understand the language of these plant teachers," she says, noting that she's witnessed people's lives turned upside down by their improper or misguided use. "Not everybody has to take it to benefit from the knowledge that comes through it. Seek out the people who know and get as many answers as you can. Make psychedelics your last option, because your safety, your security, your spirituality is your own."

How Mescaline Works

THE CLASSIC PSYCHEDELIC compound 3,4,5-trimethoxy-phenethylamine, better known as mescaline, occurs naturally in several varieties of cactus, including peyote. Like the other classic psychedelics, mescaline influences the 5-HT2 serotonin receptors in the brain. Mescaline is a partial agonist of two of the receptors, 5-HT2A and 5-HT2B, meaning it binds to and activates them, but not to the same degree as a full agonist would. Studies have shown that the action triggered by partial agonists like mescaline still increases the release and/or the reuptake of serotonin. The alkaloid mescaline also binds to and activates the 5-HT2C receptor, another member of the family of receptors, but as a full agonist rather than as a partial one. These three 5-HT receptor subtypes are found in different concentrations throughout the brain and body.

Beyond its effect on serotonin receptors, mescaline—a member of the phenethylamine class, with a chemical structure that resembles that of amphetamine—also stimulates dopamine receptors, though researchers have described this effect as "modest."[1] Brain imaging has also shown that mescaline increases activity among neurons.[2]

Administration, Dosing, and Effects of Mescaline

THE WAY MESCALINE is consumed depends largely on one's cactus of choice—and one's choice can be dictated by a few different things. Some cacti, like peyote, are considered vulnerable or at risk of extinction. Some contain lower concentrations of mescaline, requiring large quantities of bitter plant matter to be consumed. There are a few cacti that contain mescaline, but the two main varieties consumed by humans are peyote and San Pedro. While peyote buttons can be chewed and eaten, another common method of administration involves the preparation of an infusion or tea-like brew. (This is how the San Pedro cactus is prepared for consumption.) Concentrations of mescaline in peyote and San Pedro cacti vary widely from one cactus to the next; however, one study notes that 10 to 20 grams of dried peyote (between three and five buttons) may contain anywhere from 200 to 400 milligrams of mescaline.[3]

Because mescaline is of low potency (one study describes it as having one twentieth of the potency of psilocybin, and one two-hundredth of a dose of LSD),[4] people need to consume a significant amount to experience effects of the drug. Where a four-hour experience with psilocybin might require a dose of 20 to 40 milligrams, and an eight-to-twelve-hour experience with LSD requires just 0.05 to 0.2 milligrams, a mescaline trip exceeding ten or twelve hours in length requires a dose of anywhere from 200 to 500 milligrams.

Mescaline, a drug once described to me as "like ayahuasca, but gentler," brings about an altered state of consciousness often reported as warm, euphoric, and dreamlike. Like other psychedelics, it commonly produces feelings of bliss, unbridled joy, connection to nature, and boundlessness. One's sense of time is particularly stretched with mescaline, which is known for its incredibly long trip duration. While visual, auditory, and other sensory phenomena can occur under the influence of mescaline, they aren't as common as they might be on a psilocybin trip. Potentially negative side effects of mescaline include anxiety, increased heart rate, dizziness, increased perspiration, an upset stomach, nausea, and diarrhea.

As you'll read shortly, mescaline has for a long time challenged scientists eager to study its impact on humans, primarily because its effects have proven to be far less predictable than those of other psychedelics.

Mescaline and Sacred Cacti: Early Use

OF ALL THE PSYCHEDELICS, mescaline has the longest recorded history of human use. It is most notably contained in the small and notoriously slow-growing peyote cactus (*Lophophora williamsii*), and occurs in faster-growing, columnar cacti including the San Pedro (*Echinopsis pachanoi*) and its close relative, the Peruvian torch (*Echinopsis peruviana*), among several others. Archaeologists have traced the earliest ritual use of peyote to prehistoric sites in the Trans-Pecos region of Texas. (*Peyote* comes from the Nahuatl name *peyotl*, meaning "cocoon.") Archaeological discoveries have also been made in northeastern Mexico, dated around 3000 to 2500 BCE.[5]

As for the San Pedro cactus, which is native to regions in the Peruvian Andes and is also found in other parts of South America, including what is now Ecuador, Chile, Colombia, Bolivia, and Argentina, its ritualistic use dates back to the start of the Andean civilization, around 3000 BCE.[6] In *Mescaline: A Global History of the First Psychedelic*, author Mike Jay describes the relationship between humans and mescaline-containing cacti as "ancient, complex, intimate and reciprocal." The relationship is illustrated in carvings and statues on a temple site called Chavín de Huántar, dating back to 1200 BCE, which depict the San Pedro cactus wrapped in the claws of a fanged being.[7] Similarly, dried peyote buttons radiocarbon-dated to 4000 BCE were found at ancient rock-art sites in the Shumla caves in what is now Texas.

Spanish colonizers, including the Franciscan friar Bernardino de Sahagún around 1570[8] and the Jesuit priest Bernabé Cobo in 1653, observed ritualistic use of mescaline-containing cacti by Indigenous groups. Sahagún wrote of the peyote cactus: "Those who eat or drink it see visions either frightful or laughable ... it stimulates them and gives them sufficient spirit to fight and have neither fear, thirst nor hunger, and they say it guards them from all danger."[9] A missionary living in Peru, Cobo observed the use of San Pedro and described it as "the plant with which the Devil deceived the Indians of Peru in their paganism," one that led them to "[dream] a thousand absurdities and [believe] them as if they were true."[10]

While these observations were made at different times about different groups of people who used two vastly different varieties of cacti, the responses from colonizers to the use of mescaline-containing cacti in North, Central, and South America were similar. More often than not, their observations were shaped by the fear that cacti use threatened their own religious beliefs. They pointed out the similarities between the act of Communion in the Christian faith and the way Indigenous peoples consumed the cacti, seeing it as a perversion of their ritual. As a result of this fear, colonialists banned the use of peyote and threatened those who used it with severe punishment. This did not stop the spread of the peyote cult of the Huichol and the Tarahumara peoples, and eventually the Native Americans of the Great Plains began to use it as well.[11]

While far less is known about the use of San Pedro during this era (there exists no documentation of rituals involving the cactus before the arrival of Columbus), the inquisition in Peru did not persecute those who used it. However, over time, elements and symbolism of Christianity worked their way into the rites and rituals associated with the cactus. For example, while the Quechua people call the cactus *huachuma*, the greater public came to know it as San Pedro, which translates to "Saint Peter," the name of Catholicism's patron saint of rain and the keeper of the keys to heaven. The phenomenon of Christianization occurred among Indigenous groups in Central America and, later, Native Americans who used peyote, thanks to the Catholic influence of the Spanish colonizers.[12] Both cactus varieties are still used in ceremonial contexts throughout North, Central, and South America—in North America as a sacrament among members of the Native American Church (and, in some cases, outside of this context), and in Peru and throughout various regions of South America by curanderos in *mesa* (meaning "table") rituals. Historically, these rituals in Peru and surrounding areas were held in a similar context to ayahuasca ceremonies, in which a shaman drinks the medicine to diagnose illness. Today, this use has become more symbolic, and as with ayahuasca, consumption is no longer limited to curanderos or shamans.[13]

Peyote's
Introduction to Science

THE USE OF PEYOTE was introduced to scientists by the field studies authored by Smithsonian Institution ethnologist James Mooney. In 1891, Mooney became the first white man to be invited to participate in a peyote ceremony with a group of thirty Kiowa, Comanche, and Apache worshippers.[14]

Around this time, Native Americans across what is now the United States were forced onto reservations where they were barred from hunting and offered meagre rations, while their spiritual practices, including singing and dancing, were outlawed. In response to this oppression, a spiritual movement known as the Ghost Dance grew among the Plains peoples. Responding to the visions of a Paiute elder named Wodziwob, in which he foresaw the restoration and renewal of traditional ways of life and a retreat of European settlers, American forces perceived the Ghost Dance as a threat because it rejected all aspects of assimilation. Other Indigenous communities latched on to what came to be known as the "peyote religion." Historians believe that peyote was first introduced to the Native Americans living on the Plains when Comanche chief Quanah Parker took it for an illness in 1884. (Peyote was likely recommended to him by one of his wives, a Lipan Apache, who hailed from the Trans-Pecos region in which peyote grows naturally.)[15] The simultaneous opening of the Texas railroad allowed for trade among the communities living on reservations, and soon the peyote religion spread. Because of the ban on singing and dancing, ceremonies were held in tipis under the cover of night. Mooney befriended the chief, who famously said of their ceremonies, "the White man goes into his church house and talks about Jesus, but the Indian goes into his tipi and talks *to* Jesus."[16]

After he was invited to attend a peyote ceremony by a Kiowa informant, Mooney was told to "go back and tell the Whites that the Indians had a religion of their own which they loved." He honored the request, endeavoring at every opportunity to counter the forces and policies that pushed assimilation, writing journal articles, Smithsonian reports, and letters to the government. Unfortunately, his efforts did not have enough force to influence Indian agent James McLaughlin, who wrongly believed that another chief, Sitting Bull of the Hunkpapa Sioux, was responsible for promoting the Ghost Dance. McLaughlin had Sitting Bull arrested, and when a struggle ensued, officers shot him on the spot. Two weeks later, the U.S. Army carried out the massacre at Wounded Knee, where American soldiers brutally murdered close to 300 Native Americans.

Documenting how the Plains groups used peyote, Mooney wrote that they regarded the drug as "a panacea in medicine," believing it to be a cure for toothache, pain in childbirth, fever, breast pain, skin diseases, rheumatism, and alcoholism and other drug addictions, as well as diabetes, colds, and blindness.[17] He worked hard to dispel the idea among Americans that peyote and its associated spiritual practices were things to be feared. After Mooney completed his work, Quanah Parker sold him a fifty-pound sack of peyote buttons, which he took with him to Washington, D.C., and distributed to scientists at Columbian University (renamed George Washington University in 1904). There, a neurologist named Silas Weir Mitchell took part in the first scientific trials using peyote, and eventually wrote a report on his experience.[18] After reading Mitchell's report, the scientist Arthur Heffter tested the alkaloids on animals and himself, and eventually determined that mescaline was the ingredient in the peyote cactus responsible for its psychoactive properties. His research was published in 1897 and is regarded as the first study of a psychedelic compound derived from plants. Following Heffter's experiments, other scientists continued working with mescaline, and in 1919 it was synthesized by Ernst Späth.[19]

Early scientific accounts of mescaline experiences in humans varied greatly from one author to the next, but Texan physician John Raleigh Briggs's 1887 account caught the attention of scientists at the pharmaceutical company Parke-Davis: "It seemed to me my heart was simply running away with itself, and it was with considerable difficulty I could breathe air enough to keep me alive," wrote Briggs.[20] In the company's search for an alternative to cocaine, a drug that doctors had learned led to extreme dependence, peyote seemed like a reasonable alternative, and in 1893, Parke-Davis began to offer a tincture containing peyote extract as a "cardiac tonic," though it didn't take off as hoped.[21]

Heffter's accounts, on the other hand, involved "wonderful color apparitions" and dreamy visions of beaches in Italy, along with "a loss of the sense of time."[22] The experiences lasted from ten to twelve hours. In ceremonies peyote could be used consecutively over the course of two or three days, with imbibers experiencing a wave of nausea, fever, and pain before being thrust into another dimension often riddled with bright colors and sacred geometry, and providing the feeling of a warm glow.

Psychologists began to test mescaline on human subjects in the 1950s and continuing into the '60s. They saw that it was popular among artists and began to administer it to subjects in the hope of spurring some sort of emotional breakthrough. Despite the increase in case studies, reports of the drug's effects continued to vary widely from one person to the next.

Perhaps the most infamous use of mescaline occurred during World War II, when Nazis forced concentration camp prisoners to take the drug as part of an experiment that sought to determine whether it could be used as a truth serum. In the U.S., the Office of Strategic Services, a precursor to the Central Intelligence Agency, tested the drug for the same purpose. The CIA later recruited the leader of the Nazi program, Kurt Plötner, for a different program that also used psychedelic compounds in unethical ways: MK-Ultra. Running from 1953 to 1973, this top-secret program designed by the CIA sought to assess whether psychedelic drugs like mescaline and LSD could be used for mind control and brainwashing.[23] Although all documents associated with MK-Ultra were ordered to be destroyed amid the Watergate scandal of 1973, some survived. They were discovered in 1977, and later investigated in a Senate hearing following public outrage at the news that a federal agency had experimented on humans with mind-altering drugs. The profoundly unethical use of these psychedelics by Nazis and the CIA contributed to further misunderstanding of them, and likely led many people to believe that they are inherently harmful.

The Experience of Mescaline: Opening (and Closing) the Doors of Perception

ALTHOUGH MESCALINE ISN'T receiving much attention in the present day, it played a critical role in the emergence of the study of so-called psychedelic plants and compounds, and even inspired the word *psychedelic*, coined by Humphry Osmond in 1953 after he administered a synthetic version of mescaline to the British author Aldous Huxley.[24] The term comes from the Greek words *psychē*, meaning "mind" or "soul," and *dēloun*, which translates as "to make visible" or "to reveal." When Huxley published a book in 1954 describing his idyllic experience with mescaline, it permanently altered the alkaloid's reputation.

In this book, *The Doors of Perception*, Huxley touched on the origins of peyote before describing his journey with the cactus's active ingredient as "seeing what Adam had seen on the morning of his creation—the miracle, moment by moment, of naked existence."[25] Not only did Huxley describe his own experience with mescaline; he asserted the "significant fact" that the drug possibly presented a solution to the chemical imbalance thought at the time to be the cause of schizophrenia. This assertion piqued the interest of scientists, and in the 1950s psychologists tested mescaline as a treatment for schizophrenia—an idea that proved to be false—and later as a treatment for alcohol use disorder.

Unfortunately, mescaline's potential was hampered by a new drug that had recently been introduced to the world. To both the medical community and the hippies, it seemed to provide effects similar to mescaline's but in a far more efficient way. It required significantly smaller doses—less than a thousandth of a milligram—with fewer and less severe side effects. Its effects also didn't last as long. The drug, LSD, stole away the psychedelic spotlight, and by 1962, mescaline research had all but disappeared.

Modern Sacramental Use of Peyote: The Native American Church

AMONG THE NATIVE AMERICANS of the Plains and beyond, peyote use continued to spread across the country, culminating in the founding of the Native American Church in 1918 by Quanah Parker in Oklahoma. Today, it has more than 300,000 members. The hybrid faith ties in Indigenous wisdom and ways of knowing with elements of Christianity, though the inclusion of Christian elements varies from one group to the next. Members of the Native American Church are permitted to consume peyote without fear of prosecution for so-called illegal drug use, thanks to the Religious Freedom Restoration Act, which was amended in 1994: "The use, possession, or transportation of peyote by an [Indigenous person] for bona fide traditional ceremony purposes in connection with the practice of a traditional [Indigenous] religion is lawful, and shall not be prohibited by the United States or any state," it reads. "No [Indigenous person] shall be penalized or discriminated against on the basis of such use, possession or transportation."[26]

Sandor Iron Rope is an enrolled member of the Oglala Lakota Oyate from Pine Ridge, South Dakota, and is the president of the Native American Church of South Dakota. He has also served as the chair of the Native American Church of North America and is a fierce defender of the peyote cactus and the traditional practices that surround its use.

"Peyote is a way of life. It is like brushing your teeth, like putting on your shoes, like combing your hair. It's integrated in our lives as who we are today, as peyote people, as Indigenous people, and as the caretakers of Grandpa Peyote, of Grandma Peyote," he tells me by phone while traveling in South Dakota. "It's who we are, it's part of us ... It's vital to who we are in our church, and without it, there is no church and there is no ceremony." Iron Rope describes peyote as a teacher, a sacramental medicine viewed as a relative that has endured changes through time along with Indigenous peoples across what is now America.

As one might expect, there is some hesitation on the part of members of the Native American Church to divulge details of the sacramental use of peyote, given the trauma that has resulted from generations of forced assimilation and colonialism levied against Indigenous peoples. Iron Rope says "the peyote way" is a sensitive way of life, and while he shares openly about his own experiences, the colonial mindset has infringed upon the way peyote use is understood.

"Very little is understood from our perspective, so every Indigenous tribe is hesitant to share, because of the thought of theft. America is on stolen land, and so the whole concept of sharing for educational purposes is for the hope that people will understand the importance of preserving this way of life, of helping us heal our children," he says. "On and off the reservation, there are certain needs, and certainly historical trauma has been hindering a lot of our Native American community... I am a product of the Wounded Knee Massacre. Historical trauma is present, and we have to be able to recognize that to help heal."

The trauma Iron Rope talks about dates back to the late 1800s, before Wounded Knee, when diseases that his people weren't accustomed to were introduced to their communities, resulting in illness and death. Peyote ceremonies provided containers for healing. Today, these ceremonies continue in formats and movements that vary from one occasion to the next, and certainly from one congregation to the next, with a considerable emphasis on how the sacrament is harvested. Iron Rope is a firm believer that peyote, when spiritually harvested with prayerful intention, can be a vital tool in improving the mental health of Native Americans. He is currently working to create a culturally based ceremonial space in Pine Ridge—a project based on the Lakota abbreviation TTO, from the phrase *Tiognaka tawowakan otokahe*, meaning "the beginning of a sacred home"—so that Lakota people can attend and share in the healing that comes with the peyote ceremony.

"A lot of children come from broken homes. My parents passed when I was seven and when I was two, and my ability to get back and experience life has been all about love and nurturing," he says. "We have to correlate love and nurturing into our value systems, and TTO was created in that context." The vision is to provide Lakota teachings that will nurture and heal families and communities.

Another crucial aspect of Iron Rope's peyote advocacy work is his role as a board member of the Indigenous Peyote Conservation Initiative,[27] or IPCI, an organization focused on land access, stewardship, education, engagement, and peyote tending. "When we're talking about peyote, it's about survival," he says, recalling the effort it took to have the amendments made to the Religious Freedom Restoration Act to allow for the sacramental use of peyote.

"IPCI was created to ensure that generations to come would have a home, and so they could pray over and obtain their medicine in a healthy way," he says. These conservation efforts are a response to the misappropriation and exploitation of peyote, which Iron Rope says is occurring more frequently because of the so-called psychedelic renaissance. "I find myself being more vocal about the concerns that we have as Indigenous practitioners," he says. "We cannot overlook the connections that some of these communities have had to the medicine."

Reflecting on this psychedelic renaissance, Iron Rope says that there is much mainstream society can learn from Native Americans about the use of these powerful substances: "Corporate America is about the almighty dollar, and Indigenous perspective is about the health of the ecosystem," he says. "Almost all of our ceremonies include the elements of Mother Earth, and these ceremonies create a spiritual aura that cannot be measured by science."

Modern Sacramental Use of San Pedro: Embracing the Gray Areas

LAUREL SUGDEN IS a PhD candidate in ethnobotany at the University of British Columbia, under the guidance of anthropologist Wade Davis, and a scholar with the nonprofit research organization Usona Institute. Along with her Mestizo Peruvian partner, Josip Orlovac, she founded the Huachuma Collective in 2020, which in a more official capacity continues the work Orlovac has been doing since 1999: planting wild San Pedro cacti in the interest of sustainability. In addition to Sugden's studies of the plant, she has also cultivated a personal relationship with San Pedro spanning five years, which has taken her to Peru on several occasions. Unlike peyote or ayahuasca, she notes, San Pedro does not have a surviving Indigenous tradition.

"Colonization was very hard on the Andes and in the coast in Peru. Among the Quechua people, among the Q'eros, among the Indigenous peoples of Peru, there is not a surviving Indigenous tradition, but there is a lot of Catholicism as a result of Christian evangelism," she says. While very few Quechua people work with San Pedro, Sugden notes that the cactus does have a thriving center of use among Mestizo people along Peru's northern coast, where most practitioners who work with the medicine live in urban areas. The ritual in this environment is mixed, integrating elements of Catholicism, including saints, the Virgin Mary, God, Jesus, and the crucifix, as well as connections to Indigenous ancestors. Orlovac is one such practitioner, who has trained in the north-coast tradition of Peruvian shamanism since he was fifteen years old.

"My role in this work is doing a lot of listening and sense making, and really embracing those gray areas, and not trying to put some grand tradition on a pedestal," Sugden says. "San Pedro has proven for the last 500 years that that doesn't work."

From a spiritual perspective, Sugden says, San Pedro can awaken a sense in the user that "everything is alive, that everything is animate, that it has a spirit and a soul." This sense of animacy, she says, "is at the core of why reciprocity works the way that it does in the Andean world," where it's common for people to make offerings to the land instead of simply issuing a thought or a word of gratitude: "In our culture and modernity, it's all about 'transcending the physical'... in my own sense making, this act of providing an offering makes the relationship real. You're not grasping at an idea; you're physically showing up." This sense of physical embodiment, of oneness, and of the collective comes up repeatedly among users of San Pedro, and Sugden suggests it is, in a way, counter to the current narrative about the use of psychedelics.

"There is often this mindset of 'How can I use this for my benefit?' and San Pedro asks us the opposite: 'How are you going to be for everything else's benefit?'" This idea that San Pedro can inspire more than self-betterment is echoed by Orlovac: "The plants have taught me about freedom, about acceptance of myself, and about unconditional love," he says. "As many negative things that might be in your life, there is always an opportunity to create balance, and the plant has the compassion to show you that not all in life is lost."

Sugden and Orlovac's work through the Huachuma Collective is an extension of their offering to the cacti, which, in Orlovac's case, has been going on for more than twenty years. It currently focuses on a garden of nearly 5,000 heads of San Pedro cacti near Lima that he has cared for since 1999. In that time, he's seen wild populations of San Pedro cacti decimated by those looking to sell them to practitioners in the city of Cuzco, where, Sugden says, hundreds of people drink the bitter brew on any given night.

Case Study
Creating a Container of
Safety With San Pedro

Mary Larson (not her real name) is a plant medicine practitioner in British Columbia, Canada, who has worked with
San Pedro and a variety of other plant medicines for over a
decade. A woman who has devoted her life to creating a safe
environment in which members of her tight-knit community
can explore the depths of their own being and connection
with the earth through plants, she calls San Pedro by its
Quechua name, *huachuma* or *huachumito*. She describes it
as a fierce plant ally that can perform what she likes to call a
sort of "spiritual genetic surgery" on people who consume it.

Unlike ayahuasca, which can be more decisive in the path
it takes you on, huachuma is a gentle grandfather, Larson
says, one that provides a quiet sense of safety, a gentle
nudge, and a pat on the back, rather than a forceful push.

"It is like feeling held in the arms of San Pedro," she says.
"San Pedro has a way of coming in there like gangbusters to
make you feel safe. That energy is very healing, because not
feeling safe is really at the root of our anxiety."

In brewing and serving San Pedro, Larson has coached
people from many walks of life through preparing to sit with
the medicine. Her advice for each of them is the same: "I try to
tell them not to have expectations, but to have a more general intention to serve your highest good. Rather than trying
to play God, ask for the highest benevolent outcome," she
says. "Then huachuma does what huachuma does, which is
give you a very individualized dose of what you need. What do
you need to uncover? What do you need to heal? What do you
need to uproot?"

Attending a ceremony comes with responsibility, and so does brewing the San Pedro. Larson does not take this process lightly. When it's time to brew medicine, she cordons off the kitchen for days so her energy is not interrupted by outside forces.

"All this energy is going into the medicine, including the love and the devotion that I am embodying, and the care I put into the purification processes," she says. "It's not witchcraft, per se, but it is using codes and frequencies of the divine."

San Pedro ceremonies typically last twelve hours, making the days when they occur "a bit of an extravaganza," Larson says. The long ceremony is cushioned between a walk that allows guests to connect with nature, and a homemade meal that takes place at the end, to break the fast.

Ultimately, the unique sense of safety that San Pedro provides allows people to step into themselves in a new way, something she's witnessed time and time again during the ceremonies, which integrate song and dance.

"When people feel safe, then they can truly express themselves," Larson says. "Feeling safe is like a stepping-stone to the mission of their soul. When you feel safe, you are accepting of yourself and others, and all of our quirky ways."

What the Science Says About...

MESCALINE AND
MENTAL HEALTH

GIVEN MESCALINE'S DRAMATIC departure from the spotlight after the emergence of LSD, modern science hasn't paid attention to it to the same extent as it has to psilocybin mushrooms or MDMA. A handful of recently published papers do exist—they

are simply not to the same scientific standard as those associated with the aforementioned substances. In a 2022 study
published in the *Journal of Psychopharmacology*, the authors
consider 452 responses to a web survey asking participants
about their previous experiences with mescaline. Of the respondents, the vast majority (66 percent) had consumed San Pedro,
followed by those who had taken peyote (36 percent) and synthetic mescaline (31 percent).

Motivations for consuming mescaline included to connect with nature or to explore their spirituality (74 percent),
with almost half reporting that they used mescaline outdoors.
Respondents overwhelmingly believed that mescaline could
lead to personal and spiritual growth and enhance creative and
cognitive abilities. A total of 81 percent of participants believed
mescaline had potential in psychotherapeutic work.

Another set of questions asked respondents about the impact
of their most memorable experience with mescaline. Almost
half of them had preexisting anxiety or depression, while 20
percent had dealt with substance misuse, 17 percent suffered
from PTSD, and 17 percent struggled with alcohol misuse. Most
respondents reported that these conditions improved following
their memorable experience: 86 percent said their depression
was better, 80 percent said their anxiety was better, 76 percent said the same about their PTSD, while 68 percent and
67 percent said their substance use and alcohol use, respectively,
had lessened.

The authors suggest that, according to these self-reported
survey results, mescaline "may produce a psychedelic experience that is associated with meaningful and spiritually
significant experiences, improvements in mental health, and
has low probability for increased use and misuse."[28]

In psychedelic treatments that took place in the 1950s, mescaline was sometimes used to treat alcohol use disorder. While a handful of studies suggest psychedelics might make a good treatment for the disorder, there are no trials specifically examining how mescaline could affect it.[29]

THE
EMPATHOGEN

Empathogens include 3,4-methylenedioxymethamphetamine, better known as MDMA or "ecstasy," as well as MDA, ethylone, mephedrone, and PMA/PMMA. Only MDMA will be covered in this book, as it is currently the only one being seriously researched. Like LSD, MDMA was created in a laboratory. It is an amphetamine and a derivative of methamphetamine. What separates it from these substances is the methylenedioxy component of MDMA, which structurally resembles mescaline. This makes for effects that offer both the stimulation of an amphetamine and the hallucinogenic effects of mescaline.[1]

The word *empathogen* means "generating a state of empathy." These drugs are referred to as such because they produce psychological effects that include increased empathy and prosocial feelings,[2] behavior that prioritizes the welfare of others in ways that often involve communion, relatedness, and openness. Researchers Ralph Metzner, a psychologist, and David E. Nichols, a pharmacologist and chemist, first used the term to describe MDMA in the early 1980s. These drugs are also sometimes referred to as "entactogens," a term coined by Nichols two years later when it was pointed out to him that the original term might imply pathogenesis, or the process by which a disease develops, rather than empathy. The secondary term is meant to imply "a touching within."[3]

In most countries around the world, MDMA is a controlled substance classified as Schedule I or Class A, meaning it has high potential for abuse and no proven medical uses. In 1986, despite pushback from physicians who wanted to research its potential in therapeutic settings, MDMA was added to the UN's Convention on Psychotropic Substances, which advises that it be classified as a Schedule I substance.[4] Over the last few years, some countries have allowed exceptions, as long as they are tied to research or medical use. Thanks in large part to the work of the Multidisciplinary Association for Psychedelic Studies, MDMA was granted a breakthrough therapy designation by the U.S. FDA in 2017. This designation allows MAPS to complete phase 3 clinical trials related to the treatment of PTSD, and essentially means the FDA agrees that there may be a place for MDMA-assisted psychotherapy.[5]

5. MDMA

FROM ECSTASY
TO EMPATHY

_____

Case Study
Adding Layers to
Love and Partnership

Charley Wininger is a New York City–based psychotherapist whose practice focuses on working with couples. Dubbed "the love doctor" by the *New York Times,* he's the author of *Listening to Ecstasy: The Transformative Power of MDMA,* a memoir about the seventy-plus experiences he's had with the drug in the last twenty years—all *after* he turned fifty. Today, at age seventy-two, he says that not only has it helped permanently shift his once-melancholy perspective on life; it's served as a sort of "superglue" for his marriage to his wife, Shelley. He doesn't point to one particular experience but says that over time, MDMA has provided him with many life lessons.

Before he and Shelley embarked on their first "roll" together (the term enthusiasts sometimes use to refer to taking MDMA), Wininger tried the drug alone and decided it didn't work for him. "I had given up on it," he says of his experiences with MDMA in the '90s. "I just saw it as this hedonistic compound. I didn't know the protocols around taking it, and I ended up having some bad aftereffects." When Shelley, a former nurse who had spent her entire life avoiding drugs, asked to try MDMA with Wininger in 2001 to deepen their relationship, he decided it was worth a shot. It was his first time using MDMA in the company of another person. He went into the experience with minimal expectations, and assumed it would be "empty and meaningless," not at all anticipating the dramatic changes that eventually took place.

"It was clearly very profound for Shelley in many ways, and it delighted me that it was useful for her," Wininger tells me by Zoom from his New York apartment. "But it also delighted me that this is a medicine that is best not done alone. Some people do it alone, and they get benefit from it, but in my experience, it's best done with a group or a partner. Doing it with Shelley showed me that this could add a whole additional layer of depth, intimacy, and joy to our relationship ... we realized we could have joyful fun on this medicine, open our hearts deeper to each other, and enjoy each other's company in a way that was a revelation to us both."

One of the most crucial takeaways for Wininger, who suffers from dysthymia, was how "exceedingly good" he could feel when he was rolling.

"That I could feel such a feeling of happiness and well-being in my body, and the contrast between that and my ordinary state, led me to see that perhaps my ordinary state was not the way things had to be ... I have this somewhat depressive mental outlook, and what [my] experiences with MDMA have helped me do is recalibrate my body and chemistry to have happier, lighter, freer experiences. It helped me recalculate my cognition and get a grip on my thought process, in the same way that meditation can do for people ... you get to see that your thinking is just your thinking, it's not necessarily the truth. MDMA has taught me not to believe everything I think. It's helped me appreciate the blessings and realize that most of the things I feared in life never came to pass."

While he and his wife were already very close, Wininger says their work with MDMA has introduced new levels of joy to their relationship. "One thing MDMA has helped us do is live according to a precept that I [share with] the couples I work with, and this is: one key to happiness is to make your relationship about something bigger than itself. The most common way to do such a thing is with children... Shelley and I don't have children together, so we made our relationship about the psychedelic community, and helping to grow it," he says. For seventeen years, the Winingers have been hosting potluck dinners, gatherings, and group experiences with other "psychonauts" (a term used to refer to people who use psychedelics), something Wininger says has added a whole new dimension to their marriage.

MDMA has also had a positive impact on Wininger's clinical practice, deepening his skills of empathy for the couples that come into his Brooklyn office. "I can feel my way into and through another person's experience and really see what it's like standing in their shoes, which helps me provide a kind of atmosphere where they feel safe with me," he says. "That tends to bring down their defenses. They tend to feel safe with me, just as I feel safe when I'm rolling. It informs my practice."

How MDMA Works

DR. MATTHEW W. JOHNSON is a professor of psychiatry and behavioral sciences at Johns Hopkins University who has studied psychedelics and other drugs extensively. While much of his current work focuses on classic psychedelics including psilocybin and LSD, he has also worked with MDMA. His research has shown how MDMA purity testing services offered at concerts and raves could help keep users safe.

While MDMA shares some similarities with classic psychedelics, what sets it apart is its effect on serotonin. Unlike classic psychedelics or dissociatives, MDMA acts as an indirect serotonergic agonist, meaning it activates serotonin receptors in the brain. It binds to and blocks the serotonin receptors to prevent its reuptake, a process that recycles neurotransmitters like serotonin, increasing the amount of serotonin in the brain.

Johnson explains it in simple terms: "MDMA is a serotonin releaser, so its neurotransmission works by one cell releasing a neurotransmitter into a gap called a synapse, and the other side receiving it," he says. "You can think of it like a pitcher and a catcher in a baseball game. MDMA acts on the pitcher's side, throwing out more balls into the field between the pitcher and the catcher." In this instance, the balls in question are serotonin, "flooding the field" with the hormone that is known to promote feelings of happiness and well-being.

"MDMA ultimately affects a bunch of types of serotonin receptors by a whole lot of serotonin itself being dumped into the space between the cells, while the classic psychedelics mimic serotonin, but do something completely different to the cells on the catcher side." In addition to serotonin, MDMA triggers the release of other neurotransmitters, including dopamine and norepinephrine. Serotonin is related to mood and behavior, while dopamine is tied closely to reward, motivation, memory, and attention, and norepinephrine to stress. This increase in neurotransmitters is what leads to feelings of euphoria and increased connection to others, along with physical symptoms including increased energy, heart rate, and blood pressure.

"Ultimately, this causes it to be more stimulant-like than the classic psychedelics, which fits with its structure—it's an analogue of amphetamine and an analogue of methamphetamine," Johnson says, "but those stimulant effects have basically been tamped down [in MDMA] compared to those compounds and shifted more toward serotonin than to dopamine and norepinephrine." The release of the latter two neurotransmitters stimulates heart rate, increasing the probability of negative cardiovascular effects compared with classic psychedelics, though Johnson notes that doesn't mean the risk isn't there with the classics—just that it's relative.

Administration, Dosing, and Effects of MDMA

YOU'VE MOST LIKELY heard of MDMA as a club drug used commonly at raves, nightclubs, and music festivals, where doses and methods of administration vary. Users who purchase the drug on the illicit market primarily take it as a capsule or pressed tablet (in the latter case, pills are often pressed with mixing agents and stamped with a symbol like a happy face or a heart), but its crystalline form can also be snorted or dissolved in a liquid. Once the drug has been taken, onset generally takes anywhere from thirty to forty-five minutes, although this varies depending on dose and administration. Depending on who you ask, a "standard" dose of MDMA isn't always the same, but in research it is generally thought to be in the range of 100 to 125 milligrams, or around 1.5 milligrams per kilogram of body weight. Its effects can last from three to six hours.

"Broadly speaking on adverse effects, certainly a bad trip is more likely with a classic psychedelic," says Johnson. "It's possible with MDMA, but just like the heart risk, it's a relative difference. You're much more likely to be dealing with 'bad trip' material with classic psychedelics; people are generally having strong fear, anxiety, panicking, and that can sometimes lead to some type of harm." MDMA, on the other hand, is known more for its mood-enhancing effects that enrich the experience of recreational users at all-night raves. Those feelings of euphoria, openness, acceptance, connectedness, and lack of fear[1] resonate well in the therapy clinic, according to Johnson.

"There are a number of things about MDMA that subjectively make it a good therapeutic, and one of them is that it seems to enhance the rapport between the therapists and the participant," he says. "We know that's very important to psychotherapy, and particularly important in PTSD. There seems to be a modulation of the stress and anxiety responses. What's really needed for the treatment of PTSD is for people to be able to process their traumatic material, so they've got to talk about the thing that terrifies them. [With MDMA,] there's an emotional tone where people are still able to engage with it, but this very strong fight-or-flight reaction is dampened down. At the same time, they're not numbed out like the way they would be on alcohol or a sedative." In fact, just the opposite: many people report feeling more attuned to their emotions and their inner pathological workings and can reach a place of self-understanding and self-forgiveness.

"So often with PTSD—be it [due to] combat or sexual violence—there's self-blame, but with MDMA people are able to realize, 'No, this wasn't my fault,'" says Johnson. Overall, MDMA seems to provide a nice mix of stimulation, reducing the anxiety response and providing greater access to the traumatic memories that have kept people with PTSD in a state of fear.

"The idea is that what's happening is the same mechanism as other psychological therapies, like prolonged exposure therapy and cognitive processing therapy, except you're more likely to actually fully engage with the process because of the biological effects of the drug, and immerse yourself into it," says Johnson. "What's happening is you're pulling up these traumatic memories and working with them. Then, when you store them again, they are in fact changed."

The Origins of MDMA

MOLLY, ECSTASY, M, AND X are all common slang names for the drug officially known as 3,4-methylenedioxymethamphetamine, or MDMA. Like LSD, this lab-created psychedelic compound has an interesting history, and no lack of myths about its origin—the primary one being that the drug was first synthesized in 1912 by German pharmaceutical company Merck with the intention of creating an appetite suppressant. While Merck *was* responsible for first synthesizing MDMA, a paper published in 2006 analyzing archival documents at Merck dating back to the year it was first synthesized found that, in fact, "there were no indications for plans to develop an appetite suppressant," but rather to create hemostatic substances (to help stop bleeding). Competitor Bayer had patented a hemostatic compound called hydrastinine, and Merck chemists Walter Beckh and Otto Wolfes were keen to have a comparable compound in Merck's arsenal. They hypothesized that a methylated analogue of the compound (methylhydrastinin) would have similar effects, and with the help of fellow chemist Anton Köllisch, they developed several iterations of the analogue, all with unique chemical formulas that would allow the substances to be patentable. MDMA was one of the compounds that resulted. At the time, it was referred to as methylsafrylamin, with a patent describing the products of the synthesis as "important intermediates for the manufacturing of therapeutically effective compounds."[2] Despite the vaguely promising description, the compound was not mentioned in Merck documents again until 1927.

Fifteen years after its first synthesis, Merck chemist Max Oberlin took note of the way MDMA's structure closely resembled that of the hormones adrenaline and ephetonine. He was the first to administer pharmacological tests with MDMA. Then, in 1952, Merck chemist Albert van Schoor conducted an experiment on the compound's toxicology using flies. His was the last experiment with MDMA until 1959, when the drug was resynthesized by chemist Wolfgang Fruhstorfer, who had an interest in stimulants. It's not clear whether he ever administered the drug to humans as part of his research, and so the effects of MDMA on people would continue to be a mystery.

While the first scientific paper on MDMA was not published until 1960—a paper written in Polish describing its synthesis—other research had taken place outside of Merck. Studies on the drug's toxicology and behavioral effects using animals were commissioned by the U.S. Army in 1953 and 1954 (alongside similar examinations of compounds like mescaline), though they were not made public until 1973.[3]

Early Study and Use of MDMA

BOTH HUMAN RESEARCH and recreational use of MDMA took off in the mid-1970s. American chemist Alexander Shulgin—sometimes regarded as "the father of MDMA"—conducted work on the drug that caught the attention of psychotherapists in California, leading to a surge in the drug's popularity. Shulgin was fascinated with psychoactive substances and synthesized more than 200 compounds, testing their effects mostly on himself or colleagues.

According to Shulgin's 1991 book *PiHKAL: A Chemical Love Story* (*PiHKAL* means "Phenethylamines I Have Known and Loved"), authored with his wife, Ann, he first synthesized MDMA in 1965. Some scientists have called this timeline into question,[4] understandably because Shulgin's lab notes make no mention of self-tests conducted with the compound. (His laboratory notebook confirms that he didn't test the compound on himself until 1976.) His first article on the effects of MDMA on humans, written with David Nichols, was not published until 1978.

Shulgin and Nichols's paper suggested that there was some street use of MDMA in 1970, and subsequent papers by other authors confirmed it was officially detected in August of that year at a crime lab in Chicago, Illinois. The dance music scene may have had something to do with this: Chicago was also the birthplace of house music, where later in the decade, DJs like Frankie Knuckles were the first to blend electronic music and disco. Throughout the early 1970s, street-synthesized MDMA was seized in Tennessee, Illinois, Colorado, and Indiana, and a lab producing MDMA was raided in Ontario, Canada, in 1976, prompting politicians there to schedule the drug that same year.[5] While there's no doubt the drug was consumed recreationally, published reports of personal use are hard to find, and so it's difficult to say exactly how the drug was used in its early days. MDMA didn't suffer the same cultural baggage as LSD, at least not until the mid-'80s.

The 1978 paper by Shulgin and Nichols characterized the effects of the compound as evoking "an easily controlled altered state of consciousness with emotional and sensual overtones... that can be compared in its effect to marijuana, to psilocybin devoid of the hallucinatory components, or to low levels of MDA," a compound closely related to MDMA.[6] These effects proved to be popular among therapists in Shulgin's home state of California, and they began using the drug in their practices in late 1976, according to his 1990 paper.[7] Shulgin introduced MDMA to psychologist Leo Zeff, who had used psychedelics in conjunction with therapy before. Zeff was so blown away by the drug's potential that he came out of retirement and proceeded to discuss it with other psychotherapists. Many who worked with MDMA in this context believed it would make a great adjunct to therapy because it imbued a greater sense of trust in the therapist and seemed to encourage patients to be more talkative. Before the drug earned the street nickname "ecstasy" in 1981, therapists who administered it to their patients gave it the name "Adam," because they believed it allowed their patients to return to a state of innocence.[8]

MDMA and
Rave Culture

OUTSIDE THE THERAPY OFFICE, MDMA became popular among American university students, the LGBTQ community, and so-called "yuppies." (A 1984 article in the *San Francisco Chronicle* dubbed it "the yuppie psychedelic.")[9] They used the drug at nightclubs and raves and found it enhanced music and socializing, and appreciated that its effects were neither as strong nor as long-lasting as LSD's. A 1985 *Newsweek* article also described MDMA as the drug of choice among people identifying with the "New Age" movement. In a 2021 paper titled "Ecstasy (MDMA): A Rebellion Coherent With the System," researchers from Spain argue that recreational MDMA users "saw ecstasy as an instrument for relaxing and opening up emotionally in a world which required a continually stressful, rigid lifestyle, in what one user called 'controlled hedonism.' "[10] MDMA's rise to fame as a club drug was not limited to North America: Ibiza,

Manchester, and London saw their own rave scenes develop in the 1980s, as underground parties took place after nightclubs shut down. This, along with the scenes in American cities like Chicago and New York, marked the beginning of "rave culture," a phenomenon that in a short time spread around the world.

MDMA's rise in popularity among young people did not go unnoticed, and in 1985, after intense media scrutiny, federal officials in the U.S. placed an emergency ban on it,[11] saying that abuse of MDMA had become a nationwide problem and that it needed to be classified as a Schedule I substance. At the time, DEA administrator John C. Lawn told the Associated Press that the ban would serve as a "stopgap measure" to curb use of the drug. Other countries including the United Kingdom eventually introduced similar legislation. Rather than deterring use, banning the drug had the opposite effect, and demand for MDMA increased in the U.S. and in Europe.[12]

The Potential Risks Associated With MDMA

WHILE ALL DRUG USE comes with a certain level of risk, illicit MDMA suffers more issues with purity than do other substances mentioned in this book. When MDMA is used in a clinical trial, the drug is pure and two therapists are present with each participant to mitigate risk. Researchers closely manage mindset and setting to ensure the user's safety. Matthew Johnson doesn't recommend the illicit use of MDMA, but he says there are factors that make its recreational use either more or less risky.

"The identity of the substance is a really big deal with MDMA," he says. "Someone that has pure MDMA is going to be at less risk than someone who just scores some tablets from somebody." Drugs that have been reported as adulterants in illicit MDMA include amphetamine, cocaine, methamphetamine, ketamine, and even the opioid fentanyl, among many others. Because of these issues, recreational users sometimes test the purity of their drugs through services offered at concerts and raves, like the ones Johnson examined in his study. (Some cities, such as Vancouver, are home to purpose-built facilities where drug users can test their drugs for free.) Johnson says it's also important to know the dose you're taking. "There's been some scary data on the manufactured pills going up into really high doses—200 milligrams or larger, which is really high for MDMA. Those doses can go well past the point where the really interesting MDMA effects start, which is about 100 or 125 milligrams." Johnson also notes that frequent use of the substance can have a negative effect on the user: "There's definitely solid evidence that MDMA in the right dose and frequency can cause long-lasting changes in the serotonin system, and that may not be good. That could lead to mood issues being more emotionally dysregulated ... people that have used hundreds of times, when you look at their serotonin system, they look different." People who use MDMA frequently may experience a depleted secretion of serotonin, which can lead to changes in mood and memory.

But is that risk great enough to put a halt to ongoing research? Not according to Johnson: "I don't think there's any credible evidence that the few administrations that you see in the clinical research, that that's any risk they should stop that research at all ... there's no magic number of experiences. Using once a week is more risky than using once a month, and using once a month is more risky than using once a year. In any use, there's going to be some risk."

Johnson also points out the risks that come with the thirst MDMA can trigger. "People can get dangerously low sodium levels if they obsessively drink water. This happens sometimes because they hear the advice that drinking a lot of water is harm reduction. If they're drinking gallons of water with this idea that it's going to make them safer, it can actually be more dangerous for them."

Risks aside, Johnson is in full support of MDMA research and its potential in therapeutic settings, and says it's great to see the drug being advanced in this way. While researchers who study other psychedelic compounds can sometimes pit one psychedelic against the other, he sees them all as having similar purposes in a clinical setting.

The Second Wave of Research

SEMINAL TO THE APPROVAL of the first MDMA studies in humans in the United States was the work of MAPS founder Rick Doblin. When he founded the organization in 1986, it had been almost twenty years since the last study of a psychedelic substance. Amid MDMA's rise to popularity among therapists, he crafted an approach that he hoped would encourage politicians to reconsider their stance on psychedelic research.

When we speak, I ask him why he decided to focus so much of his attention on MDMA, rather than other substances like LSD or psilocybin.

"Why MDMA? Because it's the most gentle of all psychedelics, it's the easiest to integrate, it's the least ego-dissolving, and it's the most inherently therapeutic of all the psychedelics," he says.

"In the late '70s and early '80s, MDMA itself had revitalized the underground psychedelic therapy community, because we had this legal thing we could talk about, but also because of the incredible therapeutic potential of MDMA." Doblin asked himself two important questions: Which drug was the most likely to make it through all the resistance to psychedelic substances, and which patient population would it have to be connected to so that not only the public, but politicians, would be sympathetic?

Part of the approach of MAPS to psychedelic research and psychedelic-assisted psychotherapy has always been that therapists are more effective in treatment settings when they themselves have experienced the drug, says Doblin. While some therapists had been hesitant about combining therapy with other psychedelic drugs (and thus taking them themselves), MDMA proved to be less threatening. "There's more fear in psychiatrists and psychotherapists about psilocybin or LSD than there is about MDMA... so it seemed like that would be the drug that would most likely make it through the system."

At the time, there was heavy pushback from some medical professionals about the potential neurotoxicity associated with repeated use of MDMA, not to mention media-generated fear related to recreational use of the drug. But to Doblin, the neurotoxicity argument was just another reason to push for research.

"I knew that neurotoxicity was a problem in terms of politics, but I knew that it wasn't a real scientific problem, in the sense that, when you balanced the risks and benefits, the risks were so minimal. The neurotoxicity and brain damage argument was theoretical, and the benefits could clearly be demonstrated... and in the end I thought that would be shown to be hollow and part of the drug war narrative, exaggerating the risks." Between 1986 and 1990, the FDA rejected five different proposed protocols for MDMA studies from institutions including Harvard and the University of California, San Francisco, all based on fear of the drug's neurotoxicity.

When it came to answering the question of patient population, Doblin had a strategy: "I knew that MDMA was great for PTSD, but because of the neurotoxicity concerns and the way that research had been blocked for almost two decades, I thought there would be a need for a highly sympathetic patient population, a population for which the currently available medicines might work well with some people, but leave a large amount of people still in need of more treatments. We were seeking a large unmet medical need, and that led us to a two-pronged strategy." One group of people Doblin decided to focus on was cancer patients nearing the end of their lives, "because it would be hard for the FDA to justify the worries about neurotoxicity" in terminal patients.

"I thought, 'People are more scared of death than they are of drugs.' MDMA could be great for that," he said, noting that he's sat with several people in their last days of life and witnessed firsthand how using the drug in this context seemed to synergize with other medications: "With opiates, [MDMA] overcomes their tranquilizing effect, and it wakes people up... so they can say goodbye to their loved ones. It's just a beautiful, beautiful thing."

In July 1992, two U.S. agencies, the National Institute on Drug Abuse and the FDA, reviewed their policies on the research of so-called hallucinogenic drugs in response to pressure from organizations like MAPS and researchers like psychiatry professor Charles Grob. Experts advised that the study of these drugs in humans be permitted, and the FDA agreed as long as the research met the scientific standards laid out for other drug research.[13]

"They basically said, 'Yes, we'll open the door to psychedelics, we'll regulate it the way you regulate any other thing, but we have to start at the beginning.' So even though we had all this evidence about doses, about people who had tried it, none had been done under the FDA," recalls Doblin. The first step was a phase 1 dose-response safety study.

The FDA approved the first human trial of MDMA, a study of the treatment of pain in terminally ill cancer patients, sponsored by MAPS and led by Grob. While the results of the study were never published, scientific interest in the substance continued, though studies straddled both sides of the discussion about MDMA's safety. Many sought to prove that the drug led to more harm than good, especially after the death of Leah Betts, a young woman living in Essex, England, who died after taking an MDMA tablet shortly after her eighteenth birthday and developing hyponatremia, which occurs when the concentration of sodium in the blood falls to abnormally low levels as a result of drinking too much water—in Betts's case, about one and a half gallons in under ninety minutes. Betts was the daughter of a former police officer and her death received extensive media coverage after her family released an image of her in a coma to the press.[14] In 1997, Grob abandoned his work with MDMA to study psilocybin in end-of-life cancer patients, telling Doblin their work was "too controversial."

"Charlie had a lower risk tolerance than I did, although I would say most people do," says Doblin with a chuckle. "So I thought, 'Let's go back to PTSD.' " In 1999, MAPS received approval to study MDMA for PTSD in Spain. At this point, Doblin had already spent much time and energy discussing his ideas with veterans' affairs groups, offering to pay them for participation in studies. Despite support from therapists and psychiatrists, political leadership in the U.S. stood in the way of Doblin's goal until around 2012, when MAPS was finally successful in convincing politicians—namely, Senator Jay Rockefeller, then a member of the Senate Committee on Veterans' Affairs—that MDMA had a place in PTSD treatment, especially when it came to vets.

"It's a sympathetic patient population, with bipartisan support—which has been really important," Doblin says. "America, more than other countries, is a warlike country, and we really hold the vets on a pedestal. I felt that the narrative of the '60s psychedelic counterculture was a key part [of the resistance]. We wouldn't necessarily get over that with cancer patients, but veterans in particular would help build support."

Since that time, MAPS has grown in more ways than one, spreading to several countries around the world and founding the MAPS Public Benefit Corporation, a for-profit company owned by MAPS (a nonprofit) which, Doblin says, simply pours profit back into research efforts. Under the FDA's data-exclusivity program, which creates incentives for developing drugs that are off-patent, the first company to develop an off-patent drug for any purpose will be granted a period of limited marketing exclusivity in the United States. (Given the results of their latest phase 3 trials, which we'll cover later, it seems likely that MAPS will be the first MDMA researcher to reach this milestone.)

"Our goal," Doblin says, "is to have a million MDMA sessions in the first six years during this period of data exclusivity, with about 25,000 trained therapists."

Case Study
"What If Everything I Know About Myself Is Wrong?"

Journalist and author Nicolle Hodges likes to describe psychedelics as a bridge serving two distinct purposes: the first to take a person from one place to the next, and the second to show them the distance that needs to be traveled. Today, she believes these compounds and the role they can play in our lives are more than either clinical or recreational. When she first made the decision to use MDMA, it wasn't one she took lightly.

"I didn't use any form of drug until much later in life," says Hodges, explaining that her rationale had been tied up in her fear of the loss of control that might come with a transcendent or out-of-body experience provided by a psychedelic compound. "MDMA fell into a category in my brain as a party drug for people who went to raves, and that was so far outside of what I felt I wanted in my life. In a way, I'm glad that I didn't have access to it, or that I restricted myself from experimenting with it until later."

These experimentations with MDMA have led to at least two profound experiences in her life, the first of which came when she was in a time of great change.

"I was asking myself one simple question: 'What if everything you know about yourself is wrong?' When MDMA presented itself to me, because I was using that question as my guiding light, it felt like the right thing for me to do, because there was an intention behind my use—and because I truly believe that when you finally ask the right question, the answer will come."

Hodges describes this time as a complete burning of her life to the ground, "a kind of swiping my hand across the table" that resulted in the end of a seven-year monogamous relationship and a decision to move away from the city of her dreams and leave her career as a television reporter—something she'd thought she wanted for her entire life—to start from scratch.

"A serendipitous sequence of events guided purely by intuition led me into a group of friends who invited me to [the annual U.S. festival] Burning Man, and I felt really safe with this group. The way that I found them felt so on-the-right-path that I felt a new bravery to do things I had never done before," she says.

Hodges arrived at the desert festival in a state of sheer awe and wonder at the absurdity of it all: the art, the people, the connections, and the understanding that everyone there was part of the fabric of the environment. "Magic seems to happen in this microcosm, with a pinging and returning of karma or serendipity," she says. It wasn't long before she took MDMA.

Surrounded by old friends and new, Hodges found herself immersed in an art installation, dancing on the deck of a submarine as the sun rose, and looking on at all the people who had had a profound impact on her life—people who six months earlier had been strangers.

"It felt like my heart was outside of my body. I felt love in a way that I had never felt it before," she says. "And by love, I mean truly connected to everything and everyone, and wanting with the whole essence of my soul and being for them to feel alive, and experience life. My mind was blown that we were there together, that this sunrise was going to happen on Earth, and how lucky we were in that moment to be alive to witness it. I felt like I caught the rising sun in my ovaries—like something had truly woken up in me."

The awakening came with a release of unresolved trauma that had been trapping Hodges in past experiences. Shame and old stories that she had been carrying were swiftly burned away: "I felt like I had all of these moments in my life that were painful, that had calcified in my heart. And every time something new presented itself to me and tried to move through me, they would get snagged on these old stories. Every time I take MDMA, it's like a wave washes through me and takes away all of those snags in my heart, and I feel how I want to feel as a soul, as an entity, as love outside of a body that is infested by ego," she says.

In the end, Hodges says, it was her trust in the process that allowed her to feel rejuvenated by relinquishing control, rather than afraid of it. "I get to come back to my body, and I get to see the work, the distance that needs to be traveled. But because I felt how good it could feel, I come back with hope, hope that I can get there again, without the use of MDMA."

What the Science Says About...

MDMA FOR
PTSD

MDMA HAS BEEN STUDIED more thoroughly for PTSD than for any other condition. The latest study of the drug's efficacy in this respect made headlines in major newspapers around the world when it was published in the spring of 2021. A randomized, double-blind, placebo-controlled phase 3 study was carried out at multiple sites in the U.S., Canada, and Israel to test the efficacy and safety of MDMA-assisted therapy for the treatment of severe PTSD. A total of ninety participants received psychotherapy sessions (three sessions with the drug and nine for integration), with half of the group receiving MDMA and the other half a placebo. It's worth noting that more than 65 percent of participants had a lifetime history of SSRI use—a quality that previous literature suggests may lead to a less robust response to MDMA. This study did not exclude participants for having co-occurring conditions like depression, dissociation, alcohol or substance use issues, and childhood trauma.

Participants were administered MDMA, with a team of trained therapists present for each session. Before and two months after the completion of the sessions, symptoms were measured using two questionnaires, one to diagnose PTSD and another to test for functional impairment, meaning the limitations a subject experiences as a result of the illness. According to the results of the questionnaires on PTSD, MDMA scored higher than placebo, with 67 percent of participants in the MDMA group no longer meeting the diagnostic criteria for PTSD, compared with 32 percent in the placebo group, at the completion of the study. What's more, a third of participants in the MDMA group met the criteria for remission, compared with just 5 percent of the placebo group. Participants with depression, substance use issues, and other conditions are often resistant to treatment, but the study showed that MDMA was equally effective for them.[15]

The authors of the paper suggest that MDMA treatment "results in significant and robust attenuation of PTSD symptoms and functional impairment," and note that participants also experienced fewer depressive symptoms. They also point out that tracking suicidality among participants throughout the study showed that the use of MDMA did not increase suicidality, although one participant in the MDMA group discontinued participation in the trial when she became depressed after an experimental session, and is defined in the study as a "non-responder"—illustrating, importantly, that MDMA is not for everyone. The authors conclude that compared with current first-line pharmaceutical and behavioral therapies, MDMA psychotherapy "has the potential to dramatically transform treatment for PTSD."

Rick Doblin, a collaborator on the study, explains the results this way: "I sometimes show these slides about how PTSD changes your brain in different ways, and MDMA changes that in exactly the opposite ways. With PTSD, you have increased activity in the amygdala; you have decreased activity in the prefrontal cortex, where you think logically; you have decreased connectivity between the hippocampus and the amygdala, where we put memories into long-term storage. This is why it feels like the traumatic memory is never in the past, it's always about to happen."

MDMA, on the other hand, "does the exact opposite. Plus, it promotes oxytocin, the hormone of love, of nursing mothers, of orgasm, of connections, friendship, and that's what builds a therapeutic alliance, but it also builds new neural connections in these prosocial areas of the brain. All of these things make MDMA ideal for PTSD."

MDMA FOR
ALCOHOL USE DISORDER

A PILOT STUDY published in 2021 considered the safety and tolerability of MDMA treatment in conjunction with psychotherapy for people suffering from alcohol use disorder. Its authors hypothesize the drug may be well suited to treating alcohol and other substance use issues—just as Dr. Ben Sessa suggested in a previous paper that the capacity for the drug to "increase feelings of empathy and compassion for the self and others" may help someone with alcohol use disorder reach a state of improved self-awareness. He also suggested that MDMA's potential lies not only in improving self-awareness, but in allowing users to approach and address psychological trauma that may be linked to their problematic drinking patterns.[16]

In the pilot study, fourteen patients aged eighteen to sixty-five with alcohol use disorder were enrolled and required to complete a detox. Each participant then received two MDMA sessions, involving 187.5 milligrams of the drug per session. As with previous studies, participants received psychological support before and after their MDMA sessions, with a therapy team in place to observe and offer support. The entire course of psychotherapy ran for eight weeks.

While changes in drinking behavior were measured throughout the study and for up to nine months after participants detoxed, safety and tolerability of the treatment were the primary measures of this study. It showed significant changes in drinking habits among the majority of participants. In the four weeks leading up to detox, participants had been drinking an average of 130.6 units of alcohol per week, but at the nine-month follow-up, eleven of the fourteen participants were drinking less than 14 units of alcohol per week. This included nine participants who had remained completely abstinent from alcohol. Only three participants of the fourteen had relapsed to more than 14 units per week, with an average amount of 18.7 units per week—still a dramatic decrease in consumption compared with the measurements taken before the start of the study.

Researchers suggest that the drug's ability to increase feelings of empathy and compassion for the self and others may play a role in the participants' self-awareness, and in reducing their denial of the harms associated with such frequent use of alcohol. They conclude that while the study demonstrates such treatment can be administered safely and is well tolerated by patients with alcohol use disorder, placebo-controlled studies are necessary to identify the role MDMA plays in treatment and to rule out the possibility that the participants' success was merely the result of eight weeks of psychological support.[17]

THE
DISSOCIATIVES

Dissociative drugs are characterized by distorted sensory perceptions and feelings of disconnection or detachment, and include iboga/ibogaine and ketamine. (Others include nitrous oxide; phencyclidine, also known as PCP; and dextromethorphan, also known as DXM.)

Their ability to induce feelings of disconnection isn't the only thing they have in common: while both ketamine and ibogaine work in multiple ways in the brain, they share a mechanism involving the NMDA (*N*-methyl-D-aspartate) receptor,[1] sometimes referred to as NMDAR. Both are NMDAR antagonists, meaning they inhibit the action of the receptors. The receptors themselves respond to neurotransmitters including glutamate and glycine.[2] One of these neurotransmitters, glutamate, stands out as one of the most important aspects of the central nervous system, modulating cognition, memory, and emotions.

Drugs that act as NMDA antagonists have been studied for several different purposes in medicine, including as anticonvulsant, anesthetic, neuroprotective, and anti-addictive treatments.[3]

While ibogaine and ketamine both have dissociative qualities and are classified as such, these compounds are not limited to action on the NMDA receptor. Their specific actions will be discussed more thoroughly in the following two chapters.

While classic psychedelics and MDMA are Schedule I or Class A compounds in most jurisdictions around the world, ketamine and iboga/ibogaine are regulated differently, both from the aforementioned class and from each other, depending on one's location. Iboga and ibogaine, for example, are generally illegal or controlled in most countries, with a few exceptions. In iboga's native country, Gabon, it is regulated by the culture ministry and protected by law. It is unregulated in a handful of countries, including Costa Rica, Brazil, Mexico, and the Netherlands, where ibogaine treatment centers have become popular. In New Zealand, another popular place for ibogaine treatment centers, it is a nonapproved prescription medication that is fully legal.

Ketamine is a controlled substance but is in a class of its own in this book, as it is an approved medicine for different medical and veterinary uses (primarily as an anesthetic or analgesic). In certain countries, it can be used legally as an off-label treatment for patients who suffer from treatment-resistant depression, anxiety disorders, eating disorders, and other mental health conditions. Of course, ketamine is also widely known for its use as a recreational or "club" drug and does have a high potential for abuse.

6. Iboga

GABON'S SACRED ROOT

Case Study
The Space to Detox

"My only friend is heroin," says Adrianne Robson in a 2019 documentary called *Dosed*. Struggling with anxiety, depression, suicidal thoughts, and a substance use problem that began not long after she first used heroin at age fifteen, Robson was approached by a close friend who had heard that using psychedelics might enable her to part ways with her opioid use, which involved a dangerous mix of methadone, heroin, morphine, and fentanyl. At this point, she'd worked with therapists and tried detox centers, and while she'd been able to stave off cravings for periods of a few weeks or months at a time, nothing had ever stuck.

Desperate to move past the habit that kept her living her life as a self-described "garbage can addict" who "will do anything" to support her habit, she agreed, albeit with some hesitancy, to seek help and experiment with psychedelics, giving her friend permission to make a film documenting her story. She started with psilocybin mushrooms, but it wasn't long before Robson and her friend the filmmaker were told by underground practitioners working with a different plant medicine that she needed something much more potent than magic mushrooms to help her through the detox process. The drug they recommended comes from iboga, an African shrub used by the Bwiti religion for ceremonial purposes. In North America, iboga and its most active alkaloid, ibogaine, are known for their ability to eliminate the unbearable physical side effects that come with opioid withdrawal, including nausea, body aches, anxiety, insomnia, sweating, and fever. These side effects are often a primary reason people with opioid dependence avoid pursuing recovery.

"I was unsure about this psychedelic drug I'd never heard of," Robson tells me in an interview. Entrusting herself to an underground group led by an initiate of Bwiti, a spiritual discipline practiced in Central Africa that incorporates the use of iboga, and in the presence of a nurse, she spent twelve days at a retreat, taking two doses of the powerful alkaloid derived from this shrub native to Gabon, one week apart. In total, Robson took iboga three times: the first two times to detox, and the third time six weeks later.

"My expectations were doubtful, even up until the night before," she says. "I was hearing stories of people who had done iboga to detox and was having trouble believing I could do the same thing."

The first ceremony began around a fire, where Bwiti rituals and traditions were discussed, and each person shared their intention. Robson found herself feeling "very uncomfortable" for most of the process—even experiencing a panic attack and landing in hospital.

During her third and final experience with iboga, Robson felt as though she experienced her own death. "I know it's cliché," she says, "but in that experience I saw how precious life really is."

Although the process was scary and very much outside the comfort zone heroin had provided for her, she now relishes the healing that comes with the use of psychedelic medicines like iboga and psilocybin, even though using them can be terrifying. It has been three and a half years since she last used opioids. "Iboga gave me that space to detox. People talk about the antidepressant effects of iboga, and I definitely felt those," says Robson. In previous times when she had detoxed, a heavy depression followed acute withdrawals, and every day felt like a slog.

"Recovery is an ongoing process. It's never done. Even for people who aren't in recovery, life is about growth and development, it's an ongoing process—and psychedelics can be helpful at different times," she says.

"It's always scary, and I avoided it because you have to face some things that you really don't want to look at. But today I try to continue to do that, because for me, psychedelics have been incredibly transformative." She describes being sober for almost four years as "completely mind-blowing."

"I could never have imagined it," she says. "I never felt the freedom that I have now."

How Iboga and Ibogaine Work

DR. BERRA YAZAR-KLOSINSKI is the chief scientific officer at MAPS Public Benefit Corporation and the deputy director at MAPS and has worked with the organization for twelve years. She is the coauthor of an observational study published in 2018 that sought to examine the effects and outcomes in individuals who had undergone ibogaine treatment at legal ibogaine centers in Mexico and New Zealand. Her explanation of the drug's mechanism is based on that work, and she notes that the shrub iboga and its active chemical ibogaine, found in highest concentrations in the plant's root bark, are studied significantly less than other psychedelic compounds. They are also being studied for only one purpose: addressing substance use issues, primarily with opioids.

"Similar to some of the other psychedelics that we're also studying, there isn't just one clear mechanism of action," she says of iboga.

A 2008 paper notes that ibogaine and its metabolite or byproduct, noribogaine (what the body breaks ibogaine down into), interact with multiple binding sites in the central nervous system, including the NMDA receptor, among others, with ibogaine binding to NMDA receptors specifically more potently than the metabolite noribogaine. Noribogaine, on the other hand, is more potent than ibogaine in binding to serotonin and preventing serotonin reuptake,[1] a similarity the drug has with MDMA. (This is likely what gives the drug its antidepressant effects.) As Yazar-Klosinski notes, noribogaine also plays a critical role in breaking chemical cravings, particularly to opioids.

"Specifically, some of what we think we know is that this active metabolite noribogaine completely inhibits the opioid receptor, and thus reduces the craving for about three months after dosing." This proves to be beneficial, she says, because it creates an opening for the patient to make the necessary changes in their life (such as adjustments to their social circles) so that they can best set themselves up for success.

Administration, Dosing, and Effects of Iboga and Ibogaine

BOTH IBOGA, the dried root bark, and ibogaine, the active alkaloid in iboga, are administered orally. Among followers of Bwiti, iboga is ground into a powder and administered in capsules, or sometimes as dried chips or mixed into a tea. According to existing literature, ibogaine is generally dosed according to body weight at an average of 15 to 20 milligrams per kilogram, although this can vary. Yazar-Klosinski notes that because of the variation from clinic to clinic in the MAPS study, it was hard for her team to know for sure just how much of the active ingredient participants were getting.

"Ibogaine is less well-described in the literature at the flood doses that are used in order to disrupt opioid misuse disorders, because the altered experience extends for many, many hours, much longer than MDMA or LSD," she says. According to MAPS's preliminary observational research, she says, large or "flood" doses of ibogaine are most successful for overcoming opioid withdrawal; however, no controlled clinical trials have been conducted yet, although there have been some phase 1 studies on healthy volunteers. "A placebo-controlled phase 2 clinical trial would enable us to answer these types of questions," she says.

Ibogaine experiences are generally quite long and can last around twelve hours and up to several days, depending on how much ibogaine is taken. Treatments are sometimes administered more than once, and sometimes consecutively.

As a dissociative, ibogaine can result in feelings of disconnection from one's body, setting, and current state, but it can also cause feelings of stimulation, sometimes keeping a user awake for more than twenty-four hours. Other side effects can include numbness, sedation, hallucinations, and reduced pain sensations. Many people who have been administered iboga or ibogaine report having out-of-body or "near-death" experiences (not unlike what Adrianne Robson experienced after taking iboga).

Although the mystical experience brought on by iboga/ibogaine has not been studied as thoroughly as the experience of LSD or magic mushrooms, there is a general understanding (and clinical research to show) that the more profound and mystical the experience, the greater and more long-lasting the effects of the trip. Yazar-Klosinski shares the subjective experience of one participant who "went back to the dawn of time and relived the big bang." The outlandishness of such an experience might lead you to question its value, but it is precisely the strange content of the experience that can make space for change in a person's life.

"That level of altered experience was beneficial, because it shifted their perspective," she says. "They realized that their day-to-day habits were just maintaining unhelpful cognitive rigidity, preventing them from being able to actually take care of themselves in the way they deserve."

Iboga:
Early Use

IBOGA HAS BEEN USED for centuries by the people who inhabit its native regions. It comes from the root of a shrub called *Tabernanthe iboga*, which grows in the jungles of Central Africa, in countries including Gabon and Cameroon. The root is still used today in powerful initiation ceremonies as part of the Bwiti spiritual belief system and religion, which historians believe came into existence as a syncretic religion in the early twentieth century, but has much earlier origins. There are several different Bwiti groups and traditions, and while practices vary from one to the next, with some pairing elements of ancestral beliefs with Christian symbolism and theology,[2] the sacramental use of iboga is the common thread that ties them all together. While Bwiti is most prominent in Gabon, Bwiti temples exist in Equatorial Guinea, Cameroon, the Democratic Republic of the Congo, and the Republic of the Congo.[3]

One such group is the Missoko Bwiti, which follows the Dissumba Bwiti tradition. While there is no official written history to document the first use of iboga by humans, the story of the discovery of the root's unique characteristics is told by Mallendi, a leader and initiation master of the Ogondé branch of the Missoko, in the book *Iboga: The Visionary Root of African Shamanism*. As the story goes, a hunter living in a village in the forest was out looking for game and came across a porcupine. As it ate the root of a shrub, the hunter, Dibenga, shot the animal with a lance and returned home to eat its intestines, a meal meant to cure intestinal parasites. After heating the intestines over a fire, Dibenga ate them and went to bed. He began to feel strange and became nauseous before stepping outside and remembering the shrub the porcupine had been eating. Returning to it the following morning, he crossed the path of a group of foragers who shared with him their ways of knowing, including their use of iboga. Once he'd mastered the lessons, he returned to his home to share what he had learned.[4]

The origin story varies for different ethnic groups. The Fang, another Bwiti group, believe it was a woman who first encountered the properties of the root, after she found the bones of her deceased husband at the base of a shrub and was instructed to eat its roots to connect with his spirit.[5] These are just two of the origin stories, and should by no means be considered exhaustive. The variety in tradition, beliefs, and practices from one Bwiti group to the next cannot be overstated.

How Bwiti Groups Use Iboga

THE NOUN BWITI is derived from the word *ebweta*, meaning "to arrive, to reach, to end up at, to emerge from one spot into another,"[6] beautifully illustrating the nature of iboga's powerful transcendental properties and its centrality to Bwiti ways of knowing. There are several different rites and initiations among Bwiti groups. They have traditionally used iboga in a ceremonial setting as an initiation, or a coming-of-age tool. Some groups focus on the initiation of men; boys in their preteen years (between nine and twelve)[7] consume iboga to initiate them into manhood, preparing them to fight and hunt. Other groups focus on girls becoming women.[8] These societies are led by healers who consume iboga and are said to gain knowledge of a person's illness through divine insight. The plant medicine is consumed for a variety of other reasons: to communicate with ancestors, gain insight about the future, resolve conflict among community members, and so on. When adherents of Bwiti pass away, bereavement ceremonies are held in their honor to help guide their souls to the afterworld. In these and other types of ceremonies, which occur under cover of darkness and can last all night, instruments are played, songs are sung, prayers are offered, and dances are performed to invoke spirits, genies, and other divine beings, primarily to bring healing. Entire communities of men, women, and children attend the festivities, which can in some cases last several days and nights. Fire plays an important role in the ceremonies, and special torches made from the resin of the okoumé tree are lit throughout the evening, their smoke creating a path for the entrance of spirits to help initiates through the experience.[9]

Of course, ceremonies in which iboga is used are just one part of Bwiti tradition, and initiates must undergo stages of training over several years before they are considered experienced enough to initiate others. In Tsogo Bwiti practices, a person who initiates others is called the *kombwe* and is at the top of the community's hierarchy.[10] These practices are still alive and well among Bwiti followers today, but like those of other plant medicines in this book, at different points in history, they have been threatened by colonialism.

European Interest in Iboga and Ibogaine

IBOGA WAS FIRST MENTIONED in an English publication in 1819, where it was described as a psychoactive plant—but it wasn't officially acknowledged by science until 1889. French botanist Henri Ernest Baillon labeled the plant based on samples of the root that had been brought back to France by a navy man named Marie-Théophile Griffon du Bellay. The French colonizers had no interest in how the people of Gabon used the root—in large doses—and assumed the drug would have toxic consequences.[11] They observed its stimulant qualities in low doses but did not discover its psychoactive properties.

In 1901, two scientists, Jan Dybowski and Edouard Landrin, extracted the plant's most concentrated alkaloid and named it ibogaine. In France, it was studied as an antifatigue drug in small doses of 10 to 30 milligrams per day. The speedlike characteristic of the drug gained attention in the 1930s and 1940s, after Albert Schweitzer opened a clinic in Lambaréné, Gabon, with an interest in iboga. Beginning in the 1930s, a drug containing ibogaine was being sold as an antifatigue medication named Lambarene. Although it would make sense that the drug was named after the city in Gabon, it was actually given the name in honor of Schweitzer, who had worked with ibogaine in his clinic in Lambaréné and brought it to the French market. The drug was described as follows: "Neuromuscular stimulant, promoting cellular combustion and eliminating fatigue; recommended in cases of depression, asthenia, convalescence, infectious diseases, abnormal intellectual or physical effort in a healthy individual ... Rapid and sustained effect without subsequent depression." Lambarene was available until 1966 and was popular among athletes, who said it gave them more stamina.[12]

Unlike LSD or magic mushrooms, iboga and ibogaine did not become a part of the cultural attraction to altered states of consciousness that emerged in the 1960s, though some self-described hippies did dabble in it. (It is said that Timothy Leary wasn't a fan of iboga because it didn't come with the same "trippy" properties as the classic psychedelics.) Scientists also weren't as interested in the drug—that is, at least until the anec-dotal experiences of an American named Howard Lotsof.

In 1962, Lotsof was nineteen years old and addicted to her-oin. When a chemist friend handed him a dose of ibogaine and tried to sell him on the experience based on the alleged thirty-six-hour length of the trip, Lotsof accepted the dose but was too afraid to take it himself. Instead, he gave it to a friend, who took it and called Lotsof within the week to let him know that the mysterious drug had changed something in him: he no longer had cravings for drugs of any kind—particularly heroin. This excited Lotsof, who had been fascinated with the idea of an "anti-drug drug." With no knowledge of dosing and not even the slightest clue of the drug's use in Gabon, he set out to acquire more doses so that he could experiment with a group of friends, twenty volunteers in total, including seven regular drug users who were addicted to cocaine or heroin. At a time when psy-chedelics were still unscheduled substances and there were no rules stipulating how and to whom they could be administered, Lotsof even created a research laboratory, S&L Laboratories, so that he could order large quantities of psychedelic substances and continue his experiments.[13]

These experiments were the first "trials" using ibogaine, and although they were improvised, five of the seven participants who consumed cocaine and heroin ceased all drug use for six months after just one experience with the "new" drug. Lotsof was among them, and said that after using ibogaine he lost the desire to use heroin.[14] "Where previously I had viewed heroin as a drug which gave me comfort, I now viewed heroin as a drug which emulated death," he says in a video posted on YouTube in 2007, in which he recounts his first experience with ibogaine. "The very next thought into my mind was 'I prefer life to death.' "[15]

Lotsof traveled to the University of California at Berkeley to take part in the movement that fought racial segregation. There, he met Leo Zeff, the psychologist and pioneer of psychedelic-assisted psychotherapy. Zeff was convinced of ibogaine's efficacy and proceeded over the next handful of years to administer the drug to some 500 patients in doses of 150 to 300 milligrams as part of his investigations into the drug. While these doses weren't large enough to generate the visions sought by Bwiti adherents, he believed them to be effective for introspection.[16] Unfortunately, by 1963 law enforcement and the FDA had picked up on Lotsof's lab. A year earlier, the FDA had passed a law requiring all researchers to submit proof of efficacy before being allowed to study drug compounds, and this put an end to S&L Laboratories.[17]

Lotsof took up the fight for ibogaine again in the early '80s, working hard to bring it to the attention of scientists and pharmaceutical companies, who responded tepidly. They didn't see the potential in a drug that could help stop addiction. Though it was an uphill battle, Lotsof's persistence played a significant role in convincing a small number of scientists to give the alkaloid the study it deserved. Patients were recruited, and the first human trials took place between 1991 and 1993 in the Netherlands, where there was more interest in pursuing treatment for heroin dependence. These were brought to an abrupt halt when a patient died.[18]

Since then, tides have shifted and there has been considerably more interest in iboga and ibogaine, primarily because of its potential to interrupt opioid dependence. Considering the vast numbers of North Americans who have died as a result of opioid dependence and misuse—more than 50,000 in the United States in 2019 alone[19]—this interest makes sense, but as a Bwiti initiate explains later on, the white man's fascination with iboga as an antidrug drug only speaks to one aspect of healing contained in the powerful West African shrub.

The Potential Risks
Associated With Iboga

SOME OF THE HESITATION in the scientific community about studying iboga and ibogaine has to do with its safety profile. According to a paper published in 2021, there were thirty-three ibogaine-related deaths between 1990 and 2020; however, it notes that ibogaine-related fatalities "occurred mostly in unsafe settings without proper medical monitoring and advanced cardiac life support capabilities" (including at so-called treatment facilities).[20] There is speculation in previous studies of opioid-related fatalities that some deaths may have occurred because of the interplay between opioids and ibogaine, a risky combination because ibogaine can increase the effect of opioid toxicity.[21]

"There are some additional cardiovascular risks, potentially on the rhythms of the heart, and how far apart they are spaced," Berra Yazar-Klosinski says. "There's a concern with ibogaine that it can alter that rhythm and spacing of the heartbeat, which can lead to a really serious condition called torsades de pointes, or TDP. It's dose-dependent, so at larger doses, it's possible that the heart rhythms can be impacted." But as Yazar-Klosinski points out, many drugs possess that risk, including the current standard of treatment for opioid use disorder.

"Regular maintenance doses of methadone carry the same risk, and so for that reason, from a risk-benefit standpoint, I think ibogaine's the better option, because it's only given a few times, as opposed to every single day over many, many years."

When I ask about other potential uses of this powerful plant medicine and its primary alkaloid, Yazar-Klosinski is quick to bring up Lambarene, the iteration of ibogaine that was commercialized in France in the early 1930s: "The Lambarene example is a good one, because I think on a day-to-day basis, many people actually struggle with having certain aspects of depressive or low mood symptoms. I think that the reason Lambarene was marketed in France was exactly because ibogaine does have these other uses at lower doses. They're just not as tough of a nut to crack as opioid use disorder," she says. This likely explains why so much effort is being put into ibogaine's anti-addictive properties.

A Bwiti Initiate on the Iboga Experience

RAVEN MARIE is an iboga cofacilitator and Bwiti initiate (one who has been initiated into the Bwiti religion) living in Costa Rica, who came to work with the medicine after finding out for herself just how life-changing a ceremony with the plant medicine could be.

"I always say, 'You don't find iboga, iboga finds you,'" she says as she dives into the story of her introduction to the medicine. Today, Marie facilitates ceremonies alongside other Bwiti initiates at a retreat center in Costa Rica called Awaken Your Soul, and has been initiated into the Missoko Bwiti tradition, the more masculine tradition "focused on personal development," Marie clarifies. When we speak, she's busy planning her next trip to Africa to be initiated into the Dissumba tradition. "The first tradition of iboga was in the Dissumba tradition, and in the Dissumba tradition, iboga is called 'the queen,' " she tells me. (We both grin ear to ear at this.)

Three years earlier, Marie had been working at a large retreat center in Costa Rica where she facilitated groups from around the world. Although she always knew she'd have an experience with plant medicine at some point in her life, she didn't expect it to be iboga. While working at the retreat center, Marie learned about the sacred root from Anthony Esposito, a Bwiti initiate and the facilitator of Awaken Your Soul, who had arrived to lead a ceremony in the Bwiti tradition.

"My beautiful Bwiti brother Anthony said, 'Oh my goodness, you're obviously of African descent, come sit with the medicine.' At that point, I'd never sat with *any* medicines. There was a part of me that was very content with where I was, but I went into the ceremony and there was a very instant understanding that I had a soul agreement to work with this medicine," says Marie, whose lineage, like the plant she works with, has roots in Africa. Her first two experiences with iboga were "highly visual," with intensely powerful visions that enabled her to do two things sought by Bwiti followers. The first was to meet with her ancestors in a vision. The second, during another experience, was to diagnose a health issue. No two journeys are the same.

"Iboga is different for everyone; it really tunes to the individual," she says. "There's no such thing as a common experience, per se. Everyone's experience is different; some people get visuals, some people don't. Some people get lots of physical aches, some people don't. Some people get knocked out and they sleep all night. It shows up on all spectrums."

While the effects can vary widely, Marie emphasizes that there are core teachings that all who use iboga will experience, things she's learned cofacilitating hundreds of iboga ceremonies and sitting with the medicine herself on a regular basis.

"One of the main core teachings of iboga is always self-love, *radical* self-love, radical self-acceptance, radical self-forgiveness. That's iboga's jam. It helps us move from a victim mentality to a sense of ownership and empowered living. It really supports us in loosening the grip of our mind in order to see through a less attached scope of awareness, so that we can see that we are not our experiences."

Marie uses the analogy of a snow globe to describe the effects of a journey with iboga: the mind is the snow globe, and iboga is your hand, shaking it up. "It pulls out the trauma from the nooks and crannies, all those things we forgot about and didn't even know how they affected us," she says. "Now, the snow has to settle, and as the snow settles, that's when you really start to see the picture clearly." Many times, guests have approached Marie after a ceremony with comments like "What was that?" and "That's the craziest thing I've ever experienced" and "I don't think I got anything out of that." Soon, the confusion disappears, and over the next forty-eight hours, they are hit with a nonstop deluge of insights and aha moments about their lives.

" 'Now I understand why I do *this*,' they'll say. It's interesting to watch those moments come without everything in the way. There's a big shake-up, and then a settling, and then clarity."

Why Iboga Is About More Than Substance Use Disorder

YOU MIGHT BE THINKING, "It sounds like all these qualities lend themselves to the treatment of substance use issues," and while that might be true, Marie is quick to point out how myopic this view of iboga is.

"I've found it very fascinating when I say 'iboga' and the first word that comes up is *addiction*," she says. "To me, this is what happens when you lose the Indigenous ways of the medicine." Not incorrectly, she points out that opioid use disorder is primarily a problem among white populations, and for people to assume that this medicine grew in the jungles of Africa "just to come over to help us with our addiction problem" is not just entitled; it's another example of what happens when colonialism driven by ego gets in the way of understanding. While she doesn't deny that iboga is helpful in the realm of addiction to opiates, she says the definition of the word *addiction* in the context of iboga needs rethinking and recontextualizing.

"I see it doing beautiful work [with substance use], but it's not the totality. It's definitely not the focus and was never the original foundation of its use. It's here to help us heal our minds and help us move beyond the limitations that we carry," she says. "Addiction can be many things. We can be addicted to our trauma, we can be addicted to our stories, to food, to shopping; addiction runs very deep. Our minds are addicted to the same repetitive programming, the same thoughts, and if it was referred to and addressed from that scope of 'addiction,' then sure, but it goes so much deeper than that."

Marie notes that, running parallel to the assumption that iboga's primary use is to treat substance use disorder, the sudden surge of scientific interest in iboga, like the fresh attention being given to other compounds in this book, is the turning of a tide driven by economic interest, something that is hard to ignore when, not too long ago, these medicines were sneered at.

"Science is a very colonized way of operating," she says. "It's a very subtle way of saying, 'Your shit don't matter until we say it does. Your truth, your Indigenous ways mean nothing until we say it does.' Some people need that scientific foundation before they can say yes to something, and I get that. It's a very interesting relationship that happens between the spiritual and the scientific, and I believe there's a place for both. I love science, and it's necessary, but science also needs to humble itself too."

Speaking to the classification of iboga as a Schedule I substance with a "high potential for abuse," Marie doesn't mince words: "The interesting thing about addiction is that the whole point is to escape something. You want to escape your reality, you want to escape your pain, you want to escape your sadness. When you take iboga, there's no escaping anything," she says. "Iboga is you, piled on top of you. It's an avalanche of you, and there is nowhere to go. This is how I know that whoever decided iboga was a Schedule I substance never actually took the medicine."

Case Study
Seeing Illness With Iboga

In March 2019, while continuing her work as a cofacilitator at Awaken Your Soul's just-opened property, Raven Marie began to feel ill throughout her entire body.

"I was feeling really tired, very low in energy. Things that were very easy for me to do were feeling incredibly challenging," she says. "At the same time, I couldn't understand why it was that I was beginning to swell up around my belly. At first, I thought maybe it was because I had been snacking too much."

Not long after, Marie felt called to sit with iboga. Working with another facilitator, they began to move through a dialogue that happens with each guest at the retreat center, in which the facilitator helps guide the guest through the experience based on what comes up.

"It's kind of like going down the rabbit hole and picking up bread crumbs along the way to understand different layers of trauma, moments of impact, and recognizing information that's long been hidden," she says. "It's so fascinating how our minds work, and how we hold on to these moments that hurt us."

Diving headfirst into the guided dialogue, Marie was told to "crawl into her belly." At first, she wasn't sure how to interpret the instruction—"How does one do that?" she thought for a moment before surrendering to the guidance.

"I crawled into my belly, and she asked, 'What do you see?' The walls of my stomach were peeling. Then, all of a sudden, everything went black, and I could see this tumor growing," remembers Marie. She felt panic in her heart. She knew that iboga sometimes delivered messages in riddles, and so she asked next, "Is this something that is happening, or something that can happen?" Iboga answered in a cheeky, soulful, singsongy voice: "It's happening!"

"Iboga has a reputation as being a very difficult or a scary medicine—and yes, it's not fun having to look at your shit, especially from a place of full ownership," she says. When she heard iboga answer her, she giggled, and knew instantly that if it was something she could laugh at, it was something she would recover from.

In the days following her journey, Marie visited a doctor, and an ultrasound confirmed that there were two fibroid tumors growing in her uterus. After two months of deep holistic work that involved addressing past trauma, microdosing with iboga, and changing her diet ("I cut out meat, dairy, eggs, and processed sugar—girl, they were all of my favorite things!"), another ultrasound confirmed that she had shrunk them down to the size of peas. Today, Marie says this deep work with iboga has helped her heal old wounds related to past relationships, as well as her relationship with her family.

"Rewriting my relationship to my trauma is what's been very profound for me. I went from absolutely being unbearably unable to spend time with my family, to now being able to receive them and love them, just as they are," she says. "Most importantly, it's allowed me to have a different relationship with myself."

What the Science Says About...

IBOGAINE AND
OPIOID USE DISORDER

ACCORDING TO A PAPER published in 2021 assessing the toxicity and therapeutic potential of ibogaine in the treatment of chronic opioid abuse, preclinical models (that is, models in animals) show that ibogaine blocks addiction-like behavior with more substances than just opioids.[22] The compound is also effective when it comes to cocaine, nicotine, and alcohol self-administration. Its authors estimate that as many as 10,000 people around the world have been treated with ibogaine based on its availability at legal clinics, as well as (illegally) online.

Clinical data that does exist on the effects of ibogaine in humans is mostly limited to the type of study Berra Yazar-Klosinski helped author: observational, or open-label, clinical trials. In the absence of more controlled trials, the information that *has* been published about ibogaine in this context has been consistent, "showing rapid resolution of opioid withdrawal symptoms, reduced cravings, and extended abstinence over weeks, often months, and sometimes years."[23]

The largest open-label study so far included two different groups of participants, 102 who were dependent on opioids, and 89 who were dependent on cocaine, with each person receiving

8 to 12 milligrams of ibogaine per kilogram of body weight—about 600 to 1,200 milligrams per person. Over 90 percent of subjects said they felt a benefit of the experience, "and that ibogaine was useful as a treatment for drug abuse"; 50 percent said they felt "cleansed" or reborn; and nearly 20 percent saw images of their death. Proving Raven Marie's point, just 16.7 percent of participants said they would be willing to undergo ibogaine treatment a second time.[24]

As Yazar-Klosinski notes, while there are existing phase 1 studies of the effects of low-dose ibogaine (just 20 milligrams) in healthy volunteers,[25] there has yet to be published clinical research on its efficacy in a randomized, placebo-controlled trial, and at the dose that's thought to be required. However, there are several studies that are either currently recruiting or have been recently green-lit by the FDA. MAPS is a collaborator in a study in Spain sponsored by the International Center for Ethnobotanical Education, Research, and Service, which will look at the safety and efficacy of ibogaine in the treatment of methadone detoxification.[26] A handful of for-profit companies are also looking at phase 1 and phase 2A trials for ibogaine and ibogaine-like drugs in the treatment of opioid use disorder.[27, 28]

"The kind of research we do is informed by real-world applications, and it really stands out compared to other kinds of drug development that I see where, typically, companies are taking a novel chemical entity and trying to figure out what it does," says Yazar-Klosinski of MAPS. "I think we tend to see overwhelmingly positive outcomes because people have been testing these medicines and these compounds on their own and anecdotally reporting what their experience is, so it's really taking this whole research pipeline and putting it on its head. We're just basically trying to prove scientifically what's already known."

7. Ketamine

DEFINITELY SPECIAL

Case Study
A Therapist in Training

Dave Phillips is a counselor who has several decades of experience as a therapist in a handful of areas, including mindfulness-based cognitive therapy, internal family systems, eye-movement desensitization and reprocessing, and relational psychotherapy. While Phillips is unable to prescribe ketamine to patients, he's certified in ketamine-assisted psychotherapy and has himself taken ketamine in a therapeutic setting about five times. He and a friend took part in a five-day ketamine training program where they were each administered two doses of ketamine on two occasions: a smaller dose administered via a lozenge, followed a few days later by a larger dose given by intramuscular injection.

Phillips's first dose made for a mild experience that he says had a "heart-opening effect," and he described himself as a chatterbox: "I felt very much in love with life, the people in my life, and I spoke about that," he says. "There were a few moments in this trip where I felt the psychedelic experience growing a little bit, and I don't always love that feeling. I struggle letting go in the psychedelic space, and so I chose not to do that."

The intramuscular dose proved to be dramatically different. "They had told us ketamine starts fast, and it really did. All of a sudden, I felt like I had just been shot out of a cannon," he recalls. "Instantly, I thought, 'I have to hold on to this.' I was on a ride, careening around all these unbelievable landscapes."

At this point in his career, Phillips had been seen as a leader in his community for a while, as one of the first to pursue work with psychedelic substances. As the roller-coaster ride he was on sped up, he felt as though his entire town was watching him.

"I could feel this energy, like, 'You can do it, Dave, you're the first one and we're following you, we're counting on you.' This has been with me my whole professional life; I like to be a leader of movements. It's what I do—I build things and I'm happy to do it ... but the longer this was going, the harder it was for me to hold on."

Phillips could feel himself disconnecting from his mind, while still feeling immense pressure to not let go. All of a sudden, as if on an amusement park ride with a dramatic change in environment, Phillips took a sharp right turn through a swirling doorway and into another scene. With a sigh of relief, he said to himself, "Thank god, I just want off this ride." And then he fell into nothingness.

Ketamine can cause amnesic effects, and so remembering an entire trip can be notoriously difficult, but what Phillips can recall he describes as "the most beautiful place I had ever been." His awareness of the outside world was nonexistent. All that existed was this place, which he says he can only accurately describe as the eternal now.

"I could have stayed there forever," he says, eyes glazing over.

Ketamine experiences of this nature generally last from forty-five minutes to an hour. Around the forty-five-minute mark, a therapist leading the group placed his hand on the back of Phillips's head and whispered into his ear. In that moment, Phillips began remembering that his friend was there—his friend, who was a human.

"Then I started becoming aware of myself, and thought, 'Hey, I think I'm a human.'" Phillips describes the next twenty minutes of reentering his body as the most beautiful part of the trip: touching his fingers together, and then to his lips, and to his arms, all the while feeling immense gratitude for his body and for the senses he was beginning to experience again. Then he remembered his wife, with whom he was about to celebrate a fortieth wedding anniversary.

"All of a sudden, we were dancing together on a lake, and there were cherry blossoms on the water," he says. "Everyone calls ketamine the strange psychedelic, and it really is, it's otherworldly... but ketamine is less about the trip, and really more about what happens later. Most of us believe that what ketamine does, is it builds resilience by giving you this experience of being separated from your thoughts... it gives you a tangible way to disconnect from them."

By disconnecting from the runaway train of pressure that his ego had placed on him, Phillips was able to integrate an important lesson about the work he was doing: "What came forward for me was to be able to say that I have more choice, that I don't have to do these things," he says. "But also, I realized the world was not against me."

How Ketamine Works

KETAMINE, SOMETIMES NICKNAMED Special K, is a synthetic drug and a dissociative anesthetic with hallucinogenic properties, available in liquid and powder forms. As a therapeutic, it can be administered intravenously, intramuscularly, orally, and nasally. Since 2011, Dr. Reid Robison has been the principal investigator and supervisor of several studies focusing on ketamine for treatment-resistant depression, including one that led to the 2019 FDA approval of esketamine (Spravato), a nasal spray intended to reduce the effects of depression and suicidal ideation. He's also a coordinating investigator with MAPS and consults on the safe use of psychedelics, and has codeveloped what's called the emotion-focused ketamine-assisted psychotherapy model, a model he uses as the medical director of an eating disorder treatment clinic in Utah called Center for Change. He says that what separates ketamine as a dissociative from classic psychedelics, including psilocybin, LSD, DMT, and mescaline, is its ability to take someone so completely out of their human existence and day-to-day reality.

"Ketamine works in a completely different way, by blocking NMDA receptors, or the glutamatergic system, rather than the serotonin system," he says. While both can induce visual hallucinations, the mystical experience is more characteristic of the classics. Unlike MDMA, ketamine is not exactly prosocial either, he says.

While ketamine is approved for use as an anesthetic, its use as a treatment for depression is off-label. More than one in five take-home prescriptions for all drugs written in the United States are as such, and Robison says this approach is necessary with certain conditions, especially for those for which there are minimal or no existing treatments. While it may only be approved as an anesthetic, ketamine was being used for depression, for example, soon after the publication of studies in 2000 by a team at Yale on the drug's antidepressant effects, which we'll learn about later in the chapter.

"Ketamine never got overscheduled like the classic psychedelics because it has this very important and commonly used role," Robison says, noting that the first time he administered it was during his residency training, when he was about to give a child stitches and wanted to help them hold still. "It's a very safe medicine that does not slow down your breathing. Psychedelics are very safe, and I would argue more so the classic psychedelics, but ketamine does have this anchor throughout history for anesthesia."

There are four distinct ways ketamine can help with severe depressive symptoms and allow someone to engage more in therapy. As an NMDA receptor blocker, it leads to a surge of glutamate release, he says, leading to rapid improvements in mood, and "waking up your neurons like you've jump-started a car battery, allowing them to communicate more freely."

Another way that ketamine works for depression, he says, was covered in a *Nature* article in 2018: ketamine turns off an antireward center in the brain known as the lateral habenula.[1] "This antireward center is overactive in stressed-out states, but ketamine quickly turns it off and reboots it, and gives you a break from this intense stress." Once that is settled down, it's easier to engage in work with a therapist.

Third, like classic psychedelics, ketamine "opens up a window of neural plasticity" where new connections can be made, and "where therapeutic work is more likely to stick." This happens because ketamine increases levels of a protein that affects brain plasticity, called the brain-derived neurotrophic factor, or BDNF.[2] BDNF plays a role in the growth and maintenance of neurons. "I would think of it as a sort of Miracle-Gro for neurons in that sense," clarifies Robison. "There's a window of opportunity you get after ketamine, where if you do a therapy session, things are more malleable and more accessible."

Finally, Robison says, ketamine interrupts the connection between the cortex and the deeper limbic system: "We might be stuck, ruminating, overthinking, having these alarm bells going off, but ketamine gives us a time-out from that. Those things can get in the way of moving through these difficult traumatic experiences and moving towards your difficult emotions ... then you can see things more clearly and go back and set up some new ways of showing up in the world."

Administration, Dosing, and Effects of Ketamine

KETAMINE COMES IN several different forms, including a clear liquid and white or off-white powder. In medical settings, it is administered in a few different ways, including via injection (intramuscular or infusion directly into a vein) and orally, although it has low oral bioavailability, meaning the drug is metabolized before it can be absorbed into the bloodstream. The effects of ketamine are entirely dose-dependent. When used in larger doses as an anesthetic, it stands out from other drugs with this purpose: where other anesthetics depress the circulatory system, ketamine stimulates it. In smaller doses, it can be used to treat pain, and in even smaller doses, it can be used in conjunction with psychotherapy to help with treatment-resistant depression. It is this last use of ketamine that is described as psychedelic, and the one that this chapter will focus on.

How ketamine is dosed depends on how it is administered: if orally, a typical dose is in the range of 200 to 300 milligrams, while an intramuscular or intravenous dose can range from 50 to 125 milligrams. How long an experience lasts is also dose- and administration-dependent: where an oral dose may provide an experience lasting between twenty minutes and one hour, intramuscular or intravenous ketamine can last longer, between forty-five and ninety minutes.

As a dissociative, ketamine can create profound feelings of detachment, and propel its users into a dreamlike state. Time and space feel distorted, while feelings of physical pain are eliminated. It can promote feelings of relaxation and joy, but it may also create confusion or nausea. Ketamine can also be addictive, and there are plenty of studies to show that repeated misuse of ketamine can lead to serious and irreversible health effects, including on the kidneys and bladder. Like MDMA, illicit ketamine may pose additional risks, especially if it is cut with other drugs.

Beyond an Anesthetic

REID ROBISON SAYS there are a few reasons ketamine is suited for use in psychotherapy settings, especially with treatment-resistant depression.

"It's a rapid antidepressant. When someone is severely depressed, it's hard to do some of the deep therapeutic work, so it's useful even outside of its psychedelic properties as a way of getting someone quickly unstuck," he says. "It gets someone out of a deep, dark place or hole or rut, so they can engage more in the work."

Other mechanisms that help with severe depressive symptoms and suicidal ideation have to do with the drug's dissociative qualities: "It gets you outside of your day-to-day, ruminating place so you can see things from a new perspective and have new insight."

Ketamine has appeal for another reason: duration. While an experience with MDMA, psilocybin, or LSD might last several hours, ketamine treatment used in psychotherapy is generally the same length as a typical therapy session, within the range of forty-five to ninety minutes. (As noted, the exact length of an experience depends on dose and how the drug is administered.) While an hour or so might feel short compared with an experience with other psychedelics, something longer might not have the same appeal to those suffering from severe depression. "When you have a six-hour experience with MDMA and a therapist present, you can get a lot accomplished," Robison says. "It's not necessarily better that it's shorter, but it makes it more accessible." He stresses, however, that the benefits of ketamine's various mechanisms may only be temporary without the crucial aspects of therapy and integration. It takes both the compound and the work outside one's experience with it for positive feelings to really stick, with the compound simply acting as a tool that allows a person to see what they are capable of.

The Origins and Recent History of Ketamine

LIKE LSD AND MDMA, the dissociative psychedelic ketamine was created in a laboratory. In the late 1950s, chemists at Parke-Davis and Company in Detroit, Michigan, were on the hunt for a compound that would act as an ideal anesthetic, while also relieving pain. Phencyclidine, or PCP, was first synthesized for this purpose in 1957. Under the name Sernyl, it was tested in animals and humans with mixed results: while it was used in surgeries, it caused increases in blood pressure and respiratory rate, and in some patients led to prolonged periods of recovery. When the medicine wore off, patients experienced extreme excitation or disturbances in behavior that involved psychotic reactions. Sometimes these effects lasted for more than twelve hours after the drug had been administered. By the end of the 1950s, it was clear that PCP was not suitable for use in humans.

In 1962, Parke-Davis chemist Calvin Lee Stevens first synthesized a derivative of phencyclidine called ketamine, named as such because the compound combined a ketone with an amine. The short-acting drug, also referred to as 2-(2-chlorophenyl)-2-(methylamino)cyclohexanone, or CI-581, was just one tenth the potency of PCP,[3] and was selected for human trials and first administered to humans in 1964. After much debate among the chemists that first worked with the drug, including Edward Domino and Guenter Corssen, ketamine, which study volunteers described as bringing a sense of "floating in outer space" and "having no feelings in the limbs,"[4] was characterized as a "dissociative" anesthetic—but not before other terms like "schizophrenomimetic" were considered. Neither Domino nor Corssen took credit for coining the term "dissociative," though—Domino credited his wife, Toni.

Ketamine was developed with the same purpose as PCP (having both anesthetic and analgesic properties), and over the years, continued study revealed that it had a higher safety profile, a shorter duration, and fewer side effects. After it was patented in Belgium in 1963, it was used as a veterinary anesthetic. (There's a reason this drug is often referred to as a horse tranquilizer.) Once it was approved for human consumption in the United States in 1970, it was used among a wide variety of patients, including children, for procedures including cardiac catheterization, skin grafts, orthopedic procedures, diagnostic procedures on the eyes, ears, nose, and throat, and minor surgical interventions.[5] It was also used as an anesthetic during the highly protested war in Vietnam, where it was preferred among medics for its fast-acting capabilities and ease of use—but its administration there did not come without problems. For some soldiers, ketamine treatment led to overuse and abuse.

In the 1980s, ketamine became popular in the electronic music scene, where it was sometimes passed off as ecstasy or MDMA, another popular drug in underground rave culture. For the next two decades, it was the illicit use of ketamine, and not its clearly defined medical purpose, that gained attention, and in 1999, the DEA classified it as a Schedule III substance.[6]

Ketamine: Medical Use and Cultural Perceptions

KETAMINE IS DESCRIBED in the scientific literature as a unique anesthetic offering a safe route to sedation, dissociation, and pain relief, with bronchodilation (the relaxing and widening of the airways, making it easier to breathe) and sympathetic nervous system stimulation (leading to the constriction of blood vessels).[7] It remains useful as a medical tool in many applications today, and is even on the World Health Organization's "Essential Medicines" list for its use as an intravenous anesthetic.

But given the different ways ketamine is perceived culturally—as mentioned earlier, as a tranquilizer for large animals, but also as a date-rape drug because of its ability to induce sedation, immobility, and amnesia—some might find it odd to see it being studied as a potential treatment for something like major depressive disorder.

It might feel brand new, but ketamine's antidepressant characteristics were first noted in the literature in 1975, when two researchers decided to evaluate its antidepressant activity. It wasn't until around the year 2000 that scientists reconsidered this area of study, but they didn't come to it through the study of depression: it was the investigation of ketamine and its influence on schizophrenia, led by John Krystal of Yale University, that resulted in further research on ketamine. The antidepressant effects of ketamine had been noted before, but the work of Krystal's team began to show how those effects were generated: by altering the body's glutamate system. This is dramatically different from the mechanism behind most antidepressants, which work with serotonin, norepinephrine, and dopamine systems. Ronald Duman, a professor of psychiatry at Yale who passed away in 2020, showed that by triggering a release of glutamate, the administration of ketamine could lead to the growth of new synapses in the brain, something that depression is known to interrupt.[8]

The Potential Risks
Associated With Ketamine

CELIA MORGAN, head of psychology and a professor of psychopharmacology at the University of Exeter, is a drug researcher who began working with ketamine during her PhD studies twenty years ago. Her work spans both the potential for improvement that can come with psychedelics, and their potential for abuse, and she has been the lead author on several studies of ketamine and other psychedelics. While she agrees that ketamine shows great promise as a treatment for depression, she recognizes that in the category of psychedelics, it isn't exactly on the same pedestal as psilocybin or MDMA for a handful of reasons.

"There's a really positive movement behind psychedelics, but I think ketamine is seen a bit like the poor, slightly dirty relative," she says. While as a clinician it's easier to work with than psilocybin or MDMA, she's troubled by its scheduling, especially when considering its safety. Although it does have a medical use, its potential for abuse is far higher than most other psychedelics. She says this is just another example of how ridiculous drug policy can be.

"I've spent quite a bit of my career researching people who struggle with using too much ketamine, and while it's not a big proportion of people, for the people it does affect, it's really serious," she says, noting that long-term side effects of problematic ketamine use are severe and can be irreversible. Chronic use can result in ketamine-induced ulcerative cystitis, sometimes referred to as ketamine bladder, which causes ulcers in the bladder that affect urination. It's a direct toxic effect of the drug that leads to the erosion of the lining of the bladder, and in severe cases a full bladder removal is required to help stop the bleeding. Morgan notes she's seen study participants as young as seventeen years old suffering from this condition, who need to use the toilet four or five times an hour.

With these risks in mind, Morgan says that ketamine's potential for abuse can be greatly reduced by the way it is presented. When embedded in therapy, the interplay between the effects of the drug and the presence of a therapist makes the experience much safer, she says. In treatment studies, there has been no evidence of patients suffering from ketamine-induced ulcerative cystitis. While her earlier work with ketamine focused on its potential for abuse, her new work involving ketamine-assisted psychotherapy for alcoholism is proving to have some promising effects.

"[These risks are] something we have to be mindful of, but my understanding of addiction is that it's not really about the drugs, it's about the person," she says. "We can demonize these drugs and not use them out of fear, or we can try and use them in treatments in a careful and conscious way."

Speaking about risks, Reid Robison points out that another thing to consider before administering the drug to a patient is their history with psychosis: if someone is predisposed to psychosis, it may induce a psychotic-type experience. This is why it's important to have careful evaluations and follow-up plans in place.

Case Study
More than a Body

Daniel Guedes is an articling law student studying the legalities of cannabis and psychedelics, and a well-versed psychedelic traveler whose physical body doesn't always agree with the drugs' side effects. When a counselor enrolled in a ketamine training program told him about ketamine and its tendency to cause dissociation from the body, he wanted to give it a try.

"I have tried out psychedelic substances before, including mushrooms, ayahuasca, DMT, LSD, and cannabis, and the onset always comes with a little bit of anxiety... it's uncomfortable, I get restless, my heart races, I breathe heavily," he says. Guedes opted to take ketamine in the context of psychotherapy and in the form of an intramuscular injection, a legal treatment option that is offered at clinics in some Canadian cities.

Ketamine was administered to Guedes in a setting created specifically for medicine sessions, while he listened to music curated for the occasion and wore eyeshades, in the presence of a medical practitioner with whom he had a trusting relationship. This, he says, is an important aspect of the ketamine experience for anyone thinking about this treatment. While the rules around ketamine administration vary from one jurisdiction to the next, advocates for psychedelic therapy encourage practitioners who administer the medicine in a clinic setting, for certain mental health conditions, to experience ketamine themselves—something that no doubt helps build trust between the therapist and the patient.

With an intention to heal and cultivate deeper connections with other people in his life, Guedes took ketamine, and said it was completely different from any previous experiences he'd had with mind-altering compounds.

"It was beyond my expectations," he says. "I couldn't feel my arms, my legs, nothing. A nothingness, as if I was a part of the universe and [my body] had dissolved. There was no ego there." Unlike mushrooms, there were no psychedelic patterns to get lost in, but he did experience synesthesia— seeing sounds—while feeling as though he was floating in the universe. Guedes also appreciated that an experience with ketamine didn't last as long as other psychedelic experiences.

"It reminded me that you are so much more than a body. You are this multidimensional being having a human experience," he says. "This is just a body, and when this body fades and passes away, your consciousness continues to live. It's eternal. We are just here having this experience in the material world, but we are so much more than this… what's the point of being anxious and worrying about things when we are so much more than our bodies, our careers, our relationships? You could say that in that moment, I experienced my true self."

While Guedes had done much personal work with psychedelics before his session, working with ketamine "was like the icing on top."

What the Science Says About...

KETAMINE AND
TREATMENT-RESISTANT DEPRESSION

ABOUT ONE THIRD of patients diagnosed with major depressive disorder don't respond to existing treatment options such as SSRIs. A patient's depression is considered to be "treatment-resistant" once they have tried at least two treatment options. As you'll recall, a pivotal study that Reid Robison was involved in led to the FDA's approval of a specific type of ketamine administered via nasal spray, called esketamine. He led the Utah site of a phase 3, open-label study that enrolled patients who then self-administered esketamine containing 14 milligrams of the active ingredient per spray. Patients dosed themselves with either 28 or 56 milligrams twice a week for four weeks, with a health-care provider present to supervise. The study demonstrated the long-term safety and tolerability of ketamine use in patients with treatment-resistant depression on a weekly or biweekly schedule, for up to one year.[9]

Many other studies that focus on ketamine and treatment-resistant depression have considered how effective the drug is when administered in different ways, via both intramuscular injection and intravenous infusion. A 2020 review of ten years of existing literature looked at the compound's efficacy when administered intravenously. It considered the results of twenty-eight studies in which subanesthetic doses of ketamine were administered to adults diagnosed with major depressive disorder, or bipolar disorder presenting with treatment-resistant depression.

Based on the analysis of data from the different studies, the authors found that 0.5 milligrams of ketamine per kilogram of body weight "was effective in reducing depression scores" in patients suffering from treatment-resistant depression. They note that the antidepressant effects of ketamine are strongest twenty-four hours after the IV infusion, when patients were six times more likely to show clinical remission than those who received a placebo. One week after treatment, that number was slightly reduced to four times.

This type of dramatic shift in mood can be critical in patients with depression, especially when they are struggling with suicidal ideation. But the review also points out that a potential downside of ketamine treatment is precisely this short-acting change: "the major challenge with ketamine is to sustain the obtained benefits which appeared to last one week after a single infusion." While some studies in the review showed that ketamine treatment can have effects lasting beyond seven days, one quarter of participants with these longer-lasting effects relapsed within seven to thirty days after receiving treatment. Like most reviews of this nature, this one concluded that more study is required to determine how effective ketamine treatment could be in the long term for patients with treatment-resistant depression.[10]

An older (but still relevant) study published in 2014 looked at the relationship between ketamine's dissociative side effects and its antidepressant effects. Administered the same dose as mentioned above, subjects in the study received ketamine by IV infusion for forty minutes. Researchers found that ketamine's dissociative side effects correlated with changes in depression more closely than its psychotomimetic or sympathomimetic (stimulation of sympathetic nerves) effects did, making dissociation a better predictor of how effective the treatment might be.[11]

While it's common to fear the sometimes unpleasant side effects that come with psychedelic experiences (in this case,

dissociation), it's reassuring to know that the precise characteristics of these compounds we tend to fear can contribute to
their efficacy.

KETAMINE AND
ALCOHOL USE DISORDER

CELIA MORGAN is currently working on studies that examine
ketamine's efficacy in people suffering from alcoholism. She
says that the dissociative qualities of ketamine support a re-
examination of self that allows people to come to new conclusions and perspectives about their use of alcohol.

"What you're asking people to do in psychological therapy
is make new connections and new perspectives, and with ketamine, the brain is in this incredibly plastic state," she says,
pointing out that patients she's interviewed in these studies describe rapid transformations after their psychedelic
experience.

"One person described taking off his alcoholic coat and hang-
ing it up during his ketamine experience and walking out a new
person," she adds.

Another aspect of ketamine that helps get to the core of a
person's alcoholism has to do with its ability to produce feelings
of connection, says Morgan: "Connection is really important in
addiction. We've reconceptualized addiction, not as anything
to do with drugs, but a disorder of connection. Having a drug
experience that allows you to tap into how you're connected to
everything around you, your place in nature, your place in the
universe—I think it's really powerful."

Another patient in one of her trials suffered abuse at the
hands of his father as a child. During his ketamine experience, Morgan says, he was able to revisit his child self with

compassion for everything that had happened in his life. The ability to observe one's life from a different perspective lends itself to therapy incredibly well. "We're using the drug to catalyze therapy, rather than giving a drug to treat something."

In the study Morgan worked on, participants took part in seven psychological therapy sessions structured around a mindfulness-based practice, and were given three infusions of ketamine. Six months after the study, they were drinking less than when the study began. While in clinical terms six months is considered quite short for a follow-up, ketamine therapy was still more successful than alternative treatments, including therapy alone. Ketamine, she says, provides an opportunity to boost plasticity in the brain, something that is reduced in individuals who drink alcohol heavily. More than that, ketamine therapy gives people with alcohol use disorder an option they didn't have before, one that represents a new kind of hope.

"For people who have tried every other treatment, it really is an amazing thing to have a bit of hope," she says. Her only worry is that the current "hype" around psychedelics might set some people up with false expectations. "We have to be careful because it's not a fit for everyone. That's the other side of it: if it doesn't work, people can become even more despondent."

Morgan was one of several authors of a recent study that looked at the safety and efficacy of ketamine to reduce relapse in patients diagnosed with alcohol use disorder. The double-blind, placebo-controlled clinical trial enrolled a total of ninety-six participants and divided them into four groups, each of which was administered a slightly different variation of treatment and placebo. The first group was given three ketamine infusions and psychological therapy, while the second received the same course of treatment with saline in place of ketamine as placebo. The third group received three ketamine infusions and alcohol education, while the fourth received saline infusions and alcohol education. Each participant attended up to ten study sessions, during which they reported any drinking events. They were also fitted with alcohol monitoring bracelets, which were attached before their infusion sessions and removed after their eighth visit, their third and final infusion. Participants were sent home with an alcohol diary to record any drinking they may have done between sessions eight and ten. During the infusion process, study participants lay on beds in a hospital room while listening to classical music through headphones, with a therapist present for support.

The results of the study showed that six months after the first infusion, participants in the ketamine groups had significantly more abstinent days than those who received the placebo. Between the two groups that received ketamine, the one that received psychological therapy had more abstinent days and lower odds of relapse than the one that received alcohol education, although the results were not statistically significant.[12]

KETAMINE AND
EATING DISORDERS

REID ROBISON'S CURRENT WORK focuses on the use of ketamine to help treat another group of conditions for which very few treatment options exist: eating disorders. He says the same mechanisms that make the drug useful in the treatment of severe depression come into play for individuals who suffer from anorexia or bulimia.

"This nonordinary state of consciousness you have on ketamine has this arc to it, so at the beginning of a ketamine experience, it's calming and there is an awareness in your body with reduced anxiety, more empathy towards self and others, and a bit of euphoria that can come with that," he says. "When I've given it to individuals with eating disorders, they often have an experience of self-love or positive body image that is rare for them, and it opens up that connection and shows them what's possible, so they can work towards accessing that more and more in day-to-day life."

Robison says the controlling thoughts that come with anorexia are like obsessive-compulsive disorder, and notes that ketamine can decrease the ego defenses that thrive on a sense of control. "As you get higher in the dose, these ego structures dissolve and you can have a complete ego dissolution and loss of identity, almost like a near-death experience... that allows someone to come back having connected to something much bigger than themselves or their eating disorder, and have a new embodied sense of knowing their worth."

Robison is currently working on a study that focuses on ketamine-assisted psychotherapy for anorexia nervosa, in which patients suffering from the eating disorder take part in psycho-therapy within twenty-four to forty-eight hours of receiving ketamine treatment, the window of time in which the mind is considered most plastic and malleable.[13] While that work is ongoing, a case series published in 2021 looking at the effects of regular intramuscular ketamine treatment in four patients with severe eating disorders and comorbid depression showed some promising results. The patients were all women who had suffered from an eating disorder and treatment-resistant depression for at least seven years, with severe, ongoing symptoms that failed to be affected by at least four antidepressant medications.

Each patient was given ketamine injections once every four to six weeks for anywhere from one year to eighteen months. The authors of this case series found that ketamine treatment reduced depression in all four women. The treatment also proved to be safe—no patients were hospitalized or required more care than what was given while the drug was administered. Two of the patients experienced "significant" changes to their illness after being stagnant in the treatment of both their disordered eating and their depression, with one showing full remission of her eating disorder and depression eighteen months after her final dose of ketamine. While the third patient in the case series experienced several personal issues that made her course of treatment more difficult (the end of a relationship and the loss of her job), she felt she was able to stay stronger and more positive in these instances than she had anticipated, in part because of the treatment. The frequency and intensity of her eating disorder behaviors were reduced, and over the course of her twelve-month treatment, her weight stabilized. Finally, the fourth patient in the case series saw some early improvements to her mood and anxiety but saw no benefit to her eating disorder symptoms.[14]

KETAMINE FOR ANXIETY AND SOCIAL ANXIETY

ALTHOUGH THERE IS less literature about ketamine's effect on anxiety than about its effect on depression, two relatively recent studies show that ketamine may have potential for some patients with anxiety and social anxiety disorders. In an uncontrolled, open-label study published in 2018, twenty patients with either generalized anxiety disorder or social anxiety disorder were administered 1 milligram of ketamine per kilogram of body weight via subcutaneous injection (not into muscle tissue, as with intramuscular injection, but into the layer of skin directly below the dermis and epidermis). This dose is described as the patient's "highest tolerated dose," and was given either once a week or twice a week, depending on the patients' responses to the ketamine treatment.

At a three-month follow-up, one quarter of the patients remained symptom-free, while one quarter "reported full re-emergence" of their symptoms within two weeks of their last dose. Eight of the twenty patients said some of the symptoms of their anxiety disorders had returned. Of the last two patients, one dropped out of the study, and the other decided to continue treatment outside the study with his doctor's help. While these numbers don't necessarily sound impressive, the paper makes clear that for those who respond to treatment, ketamine can potentially provide longer-term effects. For those who do not respond long-term, it can still provide temporary relief from symptoms; for most patients, that relief lasted for up to two weeks. This led to better ability to concentrate, improved function, and a reduction in social anxiety that allowed them "to conceptualize that they could effect changes in their lives, and this experience was empowering for them... they came to recognize that it was 'just anxiety' and that anxiety did not define who they were as people."[15]

Afterword

MOVING FORWARD MINDFULLY

———

THE PROMISE AND profound impact of psychedelics on this world cannot be denied. From their fascinating (and sometimes confusing) histories to their well-documented cultural and clinical uses, I believe that there is more than enough evidence to show that, when the variables are appropriately managed, psychedelics can be both safe and effective—not just at helping someone heal from a particular condition or ailment, but at improving outlook, open-mindedness, and overall quality of life in healthy people too.

I am hopeful that continued research will provide us with the kind of knowledge governments and medical boards need to move forward with implementing policy changes and treatment protocols to maximize the safety and efficacy of psychedelics. But I must also acknowledge and offer gratitude for the types of knowledge that exist outside scientific research: the ways of knowing belonging to the Indigenous peoples of the world who have used many of the substances mentioned in this book since time immemorial (and the knowledge keepers who generously share that information today). For too long, Indigenous ways of knowing have been disregarded by the scientific establishment, and if not disregarded, treated as though they are of little to no value. My personal experience with psychedelics has been the opposite: the more I am able to learn about a particular plant medicine before I consume it (where it came from, what it's called there, how it is traditionally used, and so on), the more gratitude I—a white Mennonite woman living in North America—have for my privilege of using it, and my experience with the substance only becomes richer. It is my reverence toward, gratitude for, and accountability to psychedelics—particularly plant medicines—that compel me to do this work. My goal with this book has been to illustrate that although the Western perspective tends to compartmentalize and silo information, psychedelics are best examined from a holistic perspective.

In looking at the current psychedelic landscape in such a way, one might notice a few roadblocks to progress. While there are many noble institutions, organizations, and companies in the emerging psychedelic field, it's clear a few perceive psychedelics as nothing more than a shiny new object on the stock market—just another vertical in which to launch a sleazy pump-and-dump scheme and take advantage of shareholders. There are also plenty of ethical questions around patenting compounds that exist in nature, compounds humans have been using, well, forever. Corporate greed and battles over intellectual property have the potential to stand in the way of the current wave of progress (as they do in every industry), and I believe both are downright antithetical to the spirit of these drugs. But then again, so is my pessimism. Things that are in the spirit of psychedelics: accountability, access, peace, love, reciprocity, and safety (just to name a few). I believe that no one comes to psychedelics without first being called to them, and I am not here to stand in anybody's way. I only hope that those with psychedelic business endeavors value what *is* in the spirit of these medicines as much as the rest of us do.

Call me naive, but I also believe that psychedelics have the potential to affect how we do business, and ultimately, how we interact with one another, thanks to their incredibly reliable ability to generate feelings of interconnectedness and empathy. By continuing to examine our relationship to psychedelics meaningfully and holding truth to power, we can build a path forward that incorporates all facets of knowledge—one paved with respect for those who came before us and hope for those who will come after us.

ACKNOWLEDGMENTS

THIS BOOK BEGAN with a note of gratitude, and it will end with one, for without the support of the people (and plants) I'm about to mention, *Psyched* would cease to exist. Let me start with an expression of thanks to the people who so generously shared their time, wisdom, understanding, and lived experience with me: trusting me with your work (whether academic or the deep inner work spurred on by a psychedelic journey) is an honor and a privilege that I do not take for granted.

To the brave individuals who were so willing to "get real" with me: Eman Salem, Daniel Carcillo, Ivy Astrix, Paul Austin, Peter Van der Heyden, Pantha Vohra, Kay Hanen, Salimeh Tabrizi, Mary Porter, Mary Larson, Charley Wininger, Nicolle Hodges, Adrianne Robson, Raven Marie, Dave Phillips, and Daniel Guedes. In every one of our conversations, I found myself so blown away by the beauty of your experiences that I struggled to form words (not a great look for an interviewer, but thank you for understanding). Your stories of healing and profound change, of willingness to trust and let go, and of moving forward with grace even when faced with immense challenges are both exemplary and unique. Thank you for helping me illustrate that no two journeys are the same, and that with the right support systems in place, even the most difficult psychedelic experiences can be prepared for and carefully integrated. Thank you for bringing color to the psychedelic experience, for sharing the deep lessons you've taken with you, and for the advice embedded in your words.

To the scientists, ethnobotanists, cultural historians, anthropologists, keepers, and advocates who said yes to my (sometimes repeated) interview requests: Dennis McKenna, Robin Carhart-Harris, Inti García Flores, Amanda Feilding, Jim Fadiman, Rick Strassman, Christopher Kilham, Zoe Helene, Bia Caiuby Labate, Sandor Iron Rope, Laurel Sugden, Josip Orlovac, Matthew Johnson, Rick Doblin, Berra Yazar-Klosinski, Reid Robison, and Celia Morgan. As journalism, my research only goes so far. It was in speaking with each of you that my research came to life. Thank you for taking the time to provide me with a level of understanding of these complex plants and compounds that could be translated to the reader. Thank you for understanding my role, and for your willingness to speak truth to power. Above all, I endeavor with every word to provide the reader with truth, and your carefully chosen words and explanations—whether scientific or cultural in nature—give shape to the historical records and research mentioned throughout this book. A special note of gratitude to Zoe Helene, who so graciously connected me with several powerful women who helped make this book what it is.

To the team at Greystone who supported my wild idea: thank you for believing that I could do these substances justice. I am especially grateful to Jennifer Croll, Brian Lynch, and Dawn Loewen for your editorial contributions. Editors are like coaches, and I'm privileged to have each of you in my corner.

To my family and my chosen family: Mom, Dad, Daniel, Keanna, little Isaac, Eric, and Honey, I know that my career path and subject of focus might be a little outside what you envisioned for me, but I'm grateful for your ability to trust in me, even when you weren't sure of the path I was on. Your guidance and advice are priceless. I hope that one day you are called to these plants, just as I was.

To the brothers and sisters whom I call friends, from the ones I've known since high school to the ones I've met in ceremony, and everyone in between: to take a psychedelic is to understand that one is not alone. Thank you for sharing in the learning of this lesson. The support and love of my community, both online and off, has truly been palpable during this experience, and on days when I wanted to give up, it's what got me through.

A few friends deserve special recognition: Wendy Shepherd, whose ability to bestow the most perfect and precise wisdom at exactly the right time will never cease to amaze me; the synchronicities in our relationship make my head spin. Miryam Lawton, whose work has so dramatically transformed my life that I can hardly remember the person I was when I first stepped into her sacred container. Salimeh Tabrizi, who recognized my passion for plant medicines several years ago and stoked that fire every step of the way, no matter how broken or unequipped I may have felt. Andrea Isaak, my ex-Menno confidant and the one who held space for me when no one else could provide me with the safety of feeling understood. Chris Bennett and Celina Archambault, whose hospitality and warmth are immeasurable and whose beautiful home in the woods provided me with the solitude and peace required to finish the final chapters of this book.

To my friends, colleagues, clients, and partners who steep themselves in the world of cannabis and psychedelics and rightly approach these medicines with the zest and zeal they deserve: I see you, I honor you, and I'm proud to stand beside you.

To the readers who support and share my stories, who have suspended their disbelief while absorbing the messages in this book, and who challenge me to write boldly: it starts and ends with you. "Thank you" doesn't really seem to cut it.

Finally, I must thank the plant medicines and lab-created compounds described in these pages. In particular, the intentional use of psilocybin mushrooms, ayahuasca, huachuma, LSD, and cannabis (very much a psychedelic) has helped bring me to a place in life where I am no longer controlled by the mental health diagnoses that turned my life upside down. Thanks to them, I feel more connected than ever to my path, my purpose in life, the people in it, and especially the world around me. I know plants and compounds can't read, but these acknowledgments would not be complete without a shout-out to the beings that guided and worked alongside me.

NOTES

INTRODUCTION

1. Maia Szalavitz, "Steve Jobs Had LSD. We Have the iPhone," *Time*, October 6, 2011, healthland.time .com/2011/10/06/jobs-had-lsd-we -have-the-iphone/

2. Nicholas Wade, "A Peek Into the Remarkable Mind Behind the Genetic Code," *New York Times*, July 11, 2006, nytimes .com/2006/07/11/science/11book .html?pagewanted=all&_r=0

3. Robert T. Gonzalez, "10 Famous Geniuses Who Basked in Recreational Drug Use," *Salon*, June 24, 2015, salon .com/2015/06/24/10_famous _geniuses_who_basked_in _recreational_drug_use/

4. Margaret Wertheim, "Pythagoras' Trousers," *Math Horizons* 3, no. 3 (February 1996): 5–7, jstor.org /stable/25678052?seq=1

5. Ralph Abraham, "Mathematics and the Psychedelic Revolution," *Multidisciplinary Association for Psychedelic Studies Newsletter* 18, no. 1 (Spring 2008): 6–8, maps .org/news-letters/v18n1/v18n1 -MAPS_8-10.pdf

6. Nathan Jeffay, "Moses Saw God 'Because He Was Stoned Again,'" *Guardian*, March 6, 2008, theguardian.com/world /2008/mar/06/religion .israelandthepalestinians

7. "The Stoned Ape," *Fantastic Fungi*, accessed April 14, 2022, fantasticfungi.com/the-mush -room/the-stoned-ape-theory/

8. Mike Jay, *Mescaline: A Global History of the First Psychedelic* (New Haven: Yale University Press, 2019), 62–65.

9. Torsten Passie and Udo Benzenhöfer, "MDA, MDMA, and Other 'Mescaline-like' Substances in the US Military's Search for a Truth Drug (1940s to 1960s)," *Drug Testing and Analysis* 10, no. 1 (January 2018): 72–80, doi.org /10.1002/dta.2292

10. Erica Dyck, "Flashback: Psychiatric Experimentation With LSD in Historical Perspective," *Canadian Journal of Psychiatry* 50, no. 7 (June 2005): 381–388, doi.org/10.1177/07067437050 5000703

11. Erika Dyck, "Psychedelic Research in 1950s Saskatchewan," *Canadian Encyclopedia*, July 16, 2019, thecanadianencyclopedia.ca/en/article/psychedelic-research-in-1950s-saskatchewan

12. R. Gordon Wasson, "Seeking the Magic Mushroom," *Life*, June 10, 1957.

13. Richard Ashley, "The Other Side of LSD," *New York Times*, October 19, 1975, nytimes.com/1975/10/19/archives/the-other-side-of-lsd.html

14. Steven J. Novak, "LSD Before Leary. Sidney Cohen's Critique of 1950s Psychedelic Drug Research," *Isis* 88, no. 1 (1997): 87–110, doi.org/10.1086/383628

15. Matthew Oram, "Efficacy and Enlightenment: LSD Psychotherapy and the Drug Amendments of 1962," *Journal of the History of Medical and Allied Sciences* 69, no. 2 (April 2014): 221–250, doi.org/10.1093/jhmas/jrs050

16. "Timothy Leary (1920–1996): The Effects of Psychotropic Drugs," *Harvard University Department of Psychology*, accessed April 14, 2022, psychology.fas.harvard.edu/people/timothy-leary

17. "The '60s Are Gone, But Psychedelic Research Trip Continues," *NPR: All Things Considered*, March 9, 2014, npr.org/2014/03/09/288285764/the-60s-are-gone-but-psychedelic-research-trip-continues

18. Benjamin T. Smith, "New Documents Reveal the Bloody Origins of America's Long War on Drugs," *Time*, August 24, 2021, time.com/6090016/us-war-on-drugs-origins/

19. "2 States in West Ban Sale of LSD; California and Nevada Act to Control Illegal Use," *New York Times*, May 31, 1966, nytimes.com/1966/05/31/archives/2-states-in-west-ban-sale-of-lsd-california-and-nevada-act-to.html

20. Jesse Jarnow, "LSD Now: How the Psychedelic Renaissance Changed Acid," *Rolling Stone*, October 6, 2016, rollingstone.com/feature/lsd-now-how-the-psychedelic-renaissance-changed-acid-115775/

21. Martin A. Lee and Bruce Shlain, *Acid Dreams: The Complete Social History of LSD: The CIA, the Sixties, and Beyond* (New York: Grove Press, 1985), 78–79.

22. Jesse Donaldson, "Hollywood Hospital: Hidden (Greater) Vancouver," *Montecristo Magazine*, April 10, 2019, montecristomagazine.com/community/new-westminster-controversial-hollywood-hospital

23. Public Law 90-639, An Act to Amend the Federal Food, Drug, and Cosmetic Act to Increase the Penalties for Unlawful Acts Involving Lysergic Acid Diethylamide (LSD) and Other Depressant and Stimulant Drugs, and for Other Purposes, October 24, 1968, uscode.house.gov/statutes/pl/90/638.pdf

24. Alexis Petridis, "How Did Alexander Shulgin Become Known as the Godfather of Ecstasy?," *Guardian*, June 3, 2014, theguardian.com/science/shortcuts/2014/jun/03/alexander-shulgin-man-did-not-invent-ecstasy-dead

25. John Rogers, "Nicholas Sand: Outlaw LSD Producer Fled to British Columbia," *Globe and Mail*, May 22, 2017, theglobeandmail.com/news/nicholas-sand-outlaw-lsd-producer-fled-to-british-columbia/article35081834/

THE CLASSIC PSYCHEDELICS

1. Matthew W. Johnson et al., "Classic Psychedelics: An Integrative Review of Epidemiology, Therapeutics, Mystical Experience, and Brain Network Function," *Pharmacology & Therapeutics* 197 (May 2019): 83–102, doi.org/10.1016/j.pharmthera.2018.11.010

2. Robin Carhart-Harris, "How Do Psychedelics Work?" *Current Opinion in Psychiatry* 32, no. 1 (January 2019): 16–21, doi.org/10.1097/YCO.0000000000000467

3. Katherine A. MacLean, Matthew W. Johnson, and Roland R. Griffiths, "Mystical Experiences Occasioned by the Hallucinogen Psilocybin Lead to Increases in the Personality Domain of Openness," *Journal of Psychopharmacology* 25, no. 11 (November 2011): 1453–1461, doi.org/10.1177/0269881111420188

CHAPTER 1

1. Michael Chary, "Psychedelic Research Finds Ego Exists in the Default Mode Network," *Gaia*, February 16, 2020, gaia.com/article/psychedelic-research-finds-ego-exists-in-the-default-mode-network

2. Gastón Guzmán, "Hallucinogenic Mushrooms in Mexico: An Overview," *Economic Botany* 62, no. 3 (November 2008): 404–412, jstor.org/stable/40390479

3. Jack Pettigrew, "Iconography in Bradshaw Rock Art: Breaking the Circularity," *Clinical and Experimental Optometry* 94, no. 5 (2011): 403–417, doi.org/10.1111/j.1444-0938.2011.00648.x

4. Marcin Andrzej Kotowski, "History of Mushroom Consumption and Its Impact on Traditional View on Mycobiota—An Example from Poland," *Microbial Biosystems* 4, no. 3 (2019): 1–13, doi.org/10.21608/MB.2019.61290

5. Cynthia Kuhn, Scott Swartzwelder, and Wilkie Wilson, *Buzzed: The Straight Facts About the Most Used and Abused Drugs from Alcohol to Ecstasy*, 4th ed. (New York: W.W. Norton, 2014), 116.

6. Carl de Borhegyi, "Breaking the Mushroom Code: Soma in the Americas: Re-opening Old Roads of Archaeological Inquiry," *Hidden in Plain Sight*, mushroomstone.com

7. R. Gordon Wasson, "Seeking the Magic Mushroom," *Life*, June 10, 1957.

8. Jerome Rothenberg, ed., *María Sabina: Selections* (Berkeley: University of California Press, 2003), 69.

9. Amanda Siebert, "An Interview With Dennis McKenna," *Inside the Jar*, November 13, 2019, insidethejar.com/an-interview-with-dennis-mckenna/

10. Roland Griffiths et al., "Psilocybin Produces Substantial and Sustained Decreases in

Depression and Anxiety in Patients With Life-Threatening Cancer: A Randomized Double-Blind Trial," *Journal of Psychopharmacology* 30, no. 12 (2016): 1181–1197, doi.org/10.1177/0269881116675513

11. Amanda Siebert, "Why Canada Could Be Next to Allow Psychedelic Therapy (And How It's Already Changing Lives)," *Forbes*, December 30, 2020, forbes.com/sites/amandasiebert/2021/12/30/why-canada-could-be-next-to-allow-psychedelic-therapy-and-how-its-already-changing-lives/?sh=69447f58eb36

12. Alan K. Davis et al., "Effects of Psilocybin-Assisted Therapy on Major Depressive Disorder: A Randomized Clinical Trial," *JAMA Psychiatry* 78, no. 5 (2021): 481–489, doi.org/10.1001/jamapsychiatry.2020.3285

13. Kuhn et al., *Buzzed*, 116.

14. Robin Carhart-Harris et al., "Trial of Psilocybin Versus Escitalopram for Depression," *New England Journal of Medicine* 384 (April 2021): 1402–1411, doi.org/10.1056/NEJMoa2032994

15. Katherine A. MacLean, Matthew W. Johnson, and Roland R. Griffiths, "Mystical Experiences Occasioned by the Hallucinogen Psilocybin Lead to Increases in the Personality Domain of Openness," *Journal of Psychopharmacology* 25, no. 11 (November 2011): 1453–1461, doi.org/10.1177/0269881111420188

16. Francisco A. Moreno et al., "Safety, Tolerability, and Efficacy of Psilocybin in 9 Patients With Obsessive-Compulsive Disorder," *Journal of Clinical Psychiatry* 67, no. 11 (November 2006), wiki.dmt-nexus.me/w/images/1/1a/psilocybin_and_ocd.pdf

17. Matthew P. Johnson et al., "Long-Term Follow-up of Psilocybin-Facilitated Smoking Cessation," *American Journal of Drug and Alcohol Abuse* 43, no. 1 (2017): 55–60, doi.org/10.3109/00952990.2016.1170135

18. Michael P. Bogenschutz et al., "Clinical Interpretations of Patient Experience in a Trial of Psilocybin-Assisted Psychotherapy for Alcohol Use Disorder," *Frontiers in Pharmacology* 9 (February 2018): article 100, doi.org/10.3389/fphar.2018.00100

CHAPTER 2

1. Stephie Grob Plante, "Meet the World's First Online LSD Microdosing Coach," *Rolling Stone*, September 7, 2017, rollingstone.com/culture/culture-features/meet-the-worlds-first-online-lsd-microdosing-coach-195817/.

2. Daniel Wacker et al., "Crystal Structure of an LSD-Bound Human Serotonin Receptor," *Cell* 168, no. 3 (2017): 377–389, doi.org/10.1016/j.cell.2016.12.033

3. "This is LSD Attached to a Brain Cell Serotonin Receptor," *UNC School of Medicine Pharmacology*, January 27, 2017, med.unc.edu/pharm/this-is-lsd-attached-to-a-brain-cell-serotonin-receptor/

4. Tom Shroder, "'Apparently Useless': The Accidental Discovery of LSD," *Atlantic*, September 9, 2014,

theatlantic.com/health/archive /2014/09/the-accidental -discovery-of-lsd/379564/

5. Albert Hofmann, *LSD: My Problem Child* (New York: McGraw-Hill, 1980), ch. 1, under "First Chemical Explorations," maps.org/images/pdf/books /lsdmyproblemchild.pdf

6. Hofmann, *LSD*, ch. 1, under "Lysergic Acid and Its Derivatives."

7. Hofmann quotations in this paragraph from *LSD*, ch. 1, under "Discovery of the Psychic Effects of LSD."

8. This and subsequent Hofmann quotations from *LSD*, ch. 1, under "Self-Experiments."

9. Mark Haden and Birgitta Woods, "LSD Overdoses: Three Case Reports," *Journal of Studies on Alcohol and Drugs* 81, no.1 (2020): 115–118, doi.org/10.15288 /jsad.2020.81.115

10. *Delysid by Sandoz, LSD-25 D-Lysergic Acid Diethylamide Tartrate* (United Kingdom: Sandoz Products Ltd., October 1964).

11. Steven J. Novak, "LSD Before Leary: Sidney Cohen's Critique of 1950s Psychedelic Drug Research," *Isis* 88, no. 1 (1997): 87–110, doi.org /10.1086/383628

12. Jesse Donaldson, "Hollywood Hospital: Hidden (Greater) Vancouver," *Montecristo Magazine*, April 10, 2019, montecristomagazine.com /community/new-westminster -controversial-hollywood-hospital

13. Novak, "LSD Before Leary."

14. David Mikkelson, "Death of Diane Linkletter," *Snopes*, August 15, 2005,

snopes.com/fact-check /the-scarlet-linkletter/

15. Sarah Sloat, "The Man Who Made It Rain Orange Sunshine," *Inverse*, January 26, 2017, inverse.com /article/26849-tim-scully-lsd -orange-sunshine-documentary -documenta

16. James Fadiman, "Microdose Research: Without Approvals, Control Groups, Double-Blinds, Staff, or Funding," *Psychedelic Press*, November 16, 2017, psychedelicpress.co.uk/blogs /psychedelic-press-blog /microdose-research-james -fadiman

17. Friederike Holze et al., "Pharmacokinetics and Pharma-codynamics of Lysergic Acid Diethylamide Microdoses in Healthy Participants," *Clinical Pharmacology & Therapeutics* 109, no. 3 (March 2021): 658–666, doi.org/10.1002/cpt.2057

18. Peter Gasser, Katharina Kirchner, and Torsten Passie, "LSD-Assisted Psychotherapy for Anxiety Associated With a Life-Threatening Disease: A Qualitative Study of Acute and Sustained Subjective Effects," *Journal of Psychopharmacology* 29, no. 1 (January 2015): 57–68, doi .org/10.1177/0269881114555249

19. Silvia Muttoni, Maddelena Ardissino, and Christopher John, "Classical Psychedelics for the Treatment of Depression and Anxiety: A Systematic Review," *Journal of Affective Disorders* 258 (November 2019): 11–24, doi .org/10.1016/j.jad.2019.07.076

20. H.A. Abramson, "LSD in Psychotherapy and Alcoholism," *American Journal of Psychotherapy* 20, no. 3 (1966): 415–438, doi.org/10.1176/appi.psychotherapy.1966.20.3.415

21. Juan José Fuentes et al., "Therapeutic Use of LSD in Psychiatry: A Systematic Review of Randomized-Controlled Clinical Trials," *Frontiers in Psychiatry* 10 (January 2020): article 943, doi.org/10.3389/fpsyt.2019.00943

22. Friederike Holze et al., "Acute Dose-Dependent Effects of Lysergic Acid Diethylamide in a Double-Blind Placebo-Controlled Study in Healthy Subjects," *Neuropsychopharmacology* 46 (2021): 537–544, doi.org/10.1038/s41386-020-00883-6

23. John C. Klock, Udo Boerner, and Charles E. Becker, "Coma, Hyperthermia and Bleeding Associated With Massive LSD Overdose," *Western Journal of Medicine* 120, no. 3 (March 1974): 183–188, ncbi.nlm.nih.gov/pmc/articles/PMC1129381/

24. Teri Krebs and Pål-Ørjan Johansen, "Lysergic Acid Diethylamide (LSD) for Alcoholism: Meta-Analysis of Randomized Controlled Trials," *Journal of Psychopharmacology* 26, no. 7 (2012): 994–1002, doi.org/10.1177/0269881112439253

25. Albert Garcia-Romeu et al., "Cessation and Reduction in Alcohol Consumption and Misuse After Psychedelic Use," *Journal of Psychopharmacology* 33, no. 9 (2019): 1088–1101, doi.org/10.1177/0269881119845793

26. Johannes G. Ramaekers et al., "A Low Dose of Lysergic Acid Diethylamide Decreases Pain Perception in Healthy Volunteers," *Psychopharmacology* 35, no. 4 (2021): 398–405, doi.org/10.1177/0269881120940937

CHAPTER 3

1. Benjamin J. Malcolm and Kelly C. Lee, "Ayahuasca: An Ancient Sacrament for Treatment of Contemporary Psychiatric Illness?" *Mental Health Clinician* 7, no. 1 (2017): 39–45, doi.org/10.9740/mhc.2017.01.039

2. Elisabet Domínguez-Clavé et al., "Ayahuasca: Pharmacology, Neuroscience and Therapeutic Potential," *Brain Research Bulletin* 26, part 1 (September 2016): 89–101, doi.org/10.1016/j.brainresbull.2016.03.002

3. Fernanda Palhano-Fontes et al., "The Psychedelic State Induced by Ayahuasca Modulates the Activity and Connectivity of the Default Mode Network," *PLoS One* 10, no. 2 (February 2015): article e0118143, doi.org/10.1371/journal.pone.0118143

4. Domínguez-Clavé, "Ayahuasca."

5. Domínguez-Clavé, "Ayahuasca."

6. Theresa M. Carbonaro and Michael B. Gatch, "Neuropharmacology of *N,N*-Dimethyltryptamine," *Brain Research Bulletin* 126, no. 1 (September 2016): 74–88, doi.org/10.1016/j.brainresbull.2016.04.016

7. Josa A. Morales-Garcia et al., "N,N-Dimethyltryptamine Compound Found in the Hallucinogenic

Tea Ayahuasca, Regulates Adult Neurogenesis in Vitro and in Vivo," *Translational Psychiatry*, 10 (2020): article 331, doi.org/10.1038 /s41398-020-01011-0

8. Daniela Peluso et al., "Reflections on Crafting an Ayahuasca Community Guide for the Awareness of Sexual Abuse," *Journal of Psychedelic Studies* 4, no. 1 (2020): 24–33, doi.org /10.1556/2054.2020.00124

9. Brian Pilecki et al., "Ethical and Legal Issues in Psychedelic Harm Reduction and Integration Therapy," *Harm Reduction Journal* 18 (April 2021): article 40, doi.org /10.1186/s12954-021-00489-1

10. Diana Quinn et al., "Addressing Abuse and Repair: An Open Letter to the Psychedelic Community," *Medium*, October 26, 2021, psychedeliccommunity .medium.com/addressing-abuse -and-repair-an-open-letter-to -the-psychedelic-community -ccf677dd92b9

11. Sachahambi, "What Indigenous Groups Traditionally Use Ayahuasca?" *Ayahuasca.com*, February 28, 2008, ayahuasca. com/psyche/shamanism/what -indigenous-groups-traditionally -use-ayahuasca/

12. Kim Kristensen, "The Ayahuasca Phenomenon—Jungle Pilgrims: North Americans Participating in Ayahuasca Ceremonies," MAPS, November 20, 2014, maps.org /articles/5408-the-ayahuasca -phenomenon

13. Melanie J. Miller et al., "Chemical Evidence for the Use of Multiple Psychotropic Plants in a 1,000-Year-Old Ritual Bundle From South America," *Proceedings of the National Academy of Sciences* 116, no. 23 (May 2019): 11207–11212, doi.org/10.1073/pnas .1902174116

14. Mark Hay, "The Colonization of the Ayahuasca Experience," JSTOR *Daily*, November 4, 2020, daily .jstor.org/the-colonization-of-the -ayahuasca-experience/

15. Luis Eduardo Luna and Steven F. White, eds., *Ayahuasca Reader: Encounters With the Amazon's Sacred Vine* (London: Synergistic, 2000), 142.

16. Beatriz Caiuby Labate and Henrik Jungaberle, eds., *The Internationalization of Ayahuasca* (Zurich: LIT Verlag, 2011), 32.

17. Villavicencio and Spruce quotations from Justin Williams, "Investigating a Century-Long Hole in History: The Untold Story of Ayahuasca from 1755-1865" (undergraduate honors thesis, University of Colorado, Boulder, 2015), core.ac.uk/download/pdf /54847411.pdf

18. Richard Evans Schultes, "The Identity of the Malpighiaceous Narcotics of South America," *Botanical Museum Leaflets, Harvard University* 18, no. 1 (1957): 1–56, jstor.org/stable/41762183

19. Williams, "Century-Long Hole."

20. Terence McKenna, *Food of the Gods: The Search for the Original Tree of Knowledge* (New York: Bantam, 1992), 24.

21. David Londoño, Jerónimo Mazarrasa, and Marc B. Aixalà, *Towards Better Ayahuasca Practices: A Guide for Organizers and Participants* (International Center for Ethnobotanical

Education, Research, and Service, 2019), 18, drogues.gencat.cat /web/.content/minisite/drogues /noticies/pdf/Guia-ayahuasca _eng_30.09.19.pdf

22. Fernanda Palhano-Fontes et al., "Rapid Antidepressant Effects of the Psychedelic Ayahuasca in Treatment-Resistant Depression: A Randomized Placebo-Controlled Trial," *Psychological Medicine* 49, no. 4 (March 2019): 655–663, doi .org/10.1017/S0033291718001356

23. Flávia de L. Osório et al., "Antidepressant Effects of a Single Dose of Ayahuasca in Patients With Recurrent Depression: A Preliminary Report," *Brazilian Journal of Psychiatry* 37, no. 1 (2015): 13–20, doi.org/10.1590/1516-4446 -2014-1496

24. Gerald Thomas et al., "Ayahuasca-Assisted Therapy for Addiction: Results From a Preliminary Observational Study in Canada," *Current Drug Abuse Reviews* 6, no. 1 (2013): 30–42, doi.org/10.2174/157339981 13099990003

25. Paulo Cesar Ribeiro Barbosa et al., "Assessment of Alcohol and Tobacco Use Disorders Among Religious Users of Ayahuasca," *Frontiers in Psychiatry* 9 (April 2018): article 136, doi.org/10.3389 /fpsyt.2018.00136

26. Simon G.D. Ruffell et al., "Ceremonial Ayahuasca in Amazonian Retreats—Mental Health and Epigenetic Outcomes From a Six-Month Naturalistic Study," *Frontiers in Psychiatry* 12 (June 2021): article 687615, doi .org/10.3389/fpsyt.2021.687615

CHAPTER 4

1. Ricardo Jorge Dinis-Oliveira, Carolina Lança Pereira, and Diana Dias da Silva, "Pharmacokinetic and Pharmacodynamic Aspects of Peyote and Mescaline: Clinical and Forensic Repercussions," *Current Molecular Pharmacology* 12, no. 3 (August 2019): 184–194, doi.org/10.2174/187446721166618 1010154139

2. Peter Kovacic and Ratnasamy Somanathan, "Novel, Unifying Mechanism for Mescaline in the Central Nervous System: Electrochemistry, Catechol Redox Metabolite, Receptor, Cell Signaling and Structure Activity Relationships," *Oxidative Medicine and Cellular Longevity* 2 (2009): article 804359, doi.org /10.4161/oxim.2.4.9380

3. Kovacic and Somanathan, "Unifying Mechanism."

4. Kovacic and Somanathan, "Unifying Mechanism."

5. Christian Rätsch, *The Encyclopedia of Psychoactive Plants: Ethnopharmacology and Its Applications* (Rochester: Park Street, 1998), 326–27.

6. Rätsch, *Encyclopedia*, 505.

7. Mike Jay, *Mescaline: A Global History of the First Psychedelic* (New Haven and London: Yale University Press, 2019), 20, 15.

8. Jay, *Mescaline*, 25.

9. Jay, *Mescaline*, 34–35.

10. Jay, *Mescaline*, 25.

11. Rätsch, *Encyclopedia*, 327–330.

12. Rätsch, *Encyclopedia*, 505–506, 329.

13. Rätsch, *Encyclopedia*, 506–507.

14. Jay, *Mescaline*, 53–75.

15. Jay, *Mescaline*, 53–75.

16. Jay, *Mescaline*, 53–75.

17. Dinis-Oliveira et al., "Pharmacokinetic and Pharmacodynamic Aspects."

18. Jay, *Mescaline*, 53–75.

19. Ivo Gurschler, "The Fourfold Discovery of Mescaline (1896–1919)," *Chemical Monthly* 150 (2019): 941–947, doi.org/10.17613/kgr6-ab31

20. Alexander S. Dawson, *The Peyote Effect: From the Inquisition to the War on Drugs* (Berkeley: University of California Press, 2018), 11.

21. Jay, *Mescaline*, 53–85.

22. Gurschler, "Fourfold Discovery."

23. Jay, *Mescaline*, 185.

24. Elaine Woo, "Humphry Osmond, 86; Coined Term 'Psychedelic,'" *Los Angeles Times,* February 22, 2004, latimes.com/archives/la-xpm-2004-feb-22-me-osmond22-story.html

25. Aldous Huxley, *The Doors of Perception* (London: Chatto & Windus, 1954), 4.

26. American Indian Religious Freedom Act Amendments of 1994, H.R. 4320, 103rd Congress (1993–94), congress.gov/bill/103rd-congress/house-bill/4230/text

27. Indigenous Peyote Conservation Initiative, ipci.life

28. Malin Vedøy Uthaug et al., "The Epidemiology of Mescaline Use: Pattern of Use, Motivations for Consumption, and Perceived Consequences, Benefits, and Acute and Enduring Subjective Effects," *Journal of Psychopharmacology* 36, no. 3 (March 2022): 309–320, doi.org/10.1177/02698811211013583

29. Michael P. Bogenshutz and Matthew W. Johnson, "Classic Hallucinogens in the Treatment of Addictions," *Progress in Neuro-Psychopharmacology and Biological Psychiatry* 64 (January 2016): 250–258, doi.org/10.1016/j.pnpbp.2015.03.002

THE EMPATHOGEN

1. Harold Kalant, "The Pharmacology and Toxicology of 'Ecstasy' (MDMA) and Related Drugs," *Canadian Medical Association Journal* 165, no. 7 (October 2001): 917–928, ncbi.nlm.nih.gov/pmc/articles/PMC81503/

2. Gillinder Bedi, David Hyman, and Harriet de Wit, "Is Ecstasy an 'Empathogen'? Effects of ±3,4-Methylenedioxymethamphetamine on Prosocial Feelings and Identification of Emotional States in Others," *Biological Psychiatry* 68, no. 12 (December 2010): 1134–1140, doi.org/10.1016/j.biopsych.2010.08.003

3. Oxford Reference, *A Dictionary of Psychology*, vol. 3, "Entactogen," oxfordreference.com/view/10.1093/oi/authority.20110803095752935

4. Nicholas Saunders, *E for Ecstasy* (self-pub., 1993), cdn.preterhuman.net/texts/literature/books_in_PDF/E%20for%20Ecstasy%20-%20Nicholas%20Saunders.pdf

5. "FDA Grants Breakthrough Therapy Designation for MDMA-Assisted Therapy for PTSD, Agrees on Special Protocol Assessment for Phase 3 Trials," MAPS, August 26, 2017, maps.org/news/media /6786-press-release-fda-grants -breakthrough-therapy -designation-for-mdma-assisted -psychotherapy-for-ptsd, -agrees-on-special-protocol -assessment-for-phase-3-trials

CHAPTER 5

1. Gillinder Bedi, David Hyman, and Harriet de Wit, "Is Ecstasy an 'Empathogen'? Effects of ±3,4-Methylenedioxy-methamphetamine on Prosocial Feelings and Identification of Emotional States in Others," *Biological Psychiatry* 68, no. 12 (December 2010): 1134–1140, doi .org/10.1016/j.biopsych.2010 .08.003

2. Roland W. Freudenmann, Florian Öxler, and Sabine Bernschneider-Reif, "The Origin of MDMA (Ecstasy) Revisited: The True Story Reconstructed From the Original Documents," *Addiction* 101 (2006): 1241–1245, doi.org/10.1111/j.1360 -0443.2006.01511.x

3. Torsten Passie and Udo Benzenhöfer, "MDA, MDMA, and Other 'Mescaline-Like' Substances in the US Military's Search for a Truth Drug (1940s to 1960s)," *Drug Testing and Analysis*, 10, no. 1 (2018): 72–80, doi.org/10.1002/dta.2292

4. Torsten Passie and Udo Benzenhöfer, "The History of MDMA as an Underground Drug in the United States, 1960–1979," *Journal of Psychoactive Drugs* 48, no. 2 (2016): 67–75, doi.org/10 .1080/02791072.2015.1128580

5. Passie and Benzenhöfer, "The History of MDMA."

6. Udo Benzenhöfer and Torsten Passie, "Rediscovering MDMA (Ecstasy): The Role of the American Chemist Alexander T. Shulgin," *Addiction* 105, no. 8 (August 2010): 1355–1361, doi.org /10.1111/j.1360-0443.2010.02948.x

7. Alexander Shulgin, "History of MDMA," in *Ecstasy: The Clinical, Pharmacological and Neurotoxicological Effects of the Drug MDMA*, ed. Stephen J. Peroutka (Boston: Kluwer Academic, 1990), 1–20.

8. "MDMA," *History*, August 21, 2018, history.com/topics/crime/history /history-of-mdma

9. José Manuel García-Montes et al., "Ecstasy (MDMA): A Rebellion Coherent With the System," *Nordic Studies on Alcohol and Drugs* 38, no. 1 (2021): 89–102, doi .org/10.1177/1455072520954329

10. García-Montes et al., "A Rebellion."

11. "U.S. Will Ban 'Ecstasy,' a Hallu-cinogenic Drug," *New York Times*, June 1, 1985, nytimes.com/1985 /06/01/us/us-will-ban-ecstasy-a -hallucinogenic-drug.html

12. García-Montes et al., "A Rebellion."

13. Rick Doblin, "The Historic FDA and NIDA Meetings on Hallucinogens," *Newsletter of the Multidisciplinary Association for Psychedelic Studies* 3, no. 3 (1992), maps.org/news-letters/vo3n3 /03302fda.html

14. "1995: Ecstasy Pill Puts Party Girl in Coma," *BBC On This Day*, news .bbc.co.uk/onthisday/hi/dates /stories/november/13/newsid _2516000/2516593.stm

15. Jennifer M. Mitchell et al., "MDMA-Assisted Therapy for Severe PTSD: A Randomized, Double-Blind, Placebo-Controlled Phase 3 Study," *Nature Medicine* 27 (May 2021): 1025–1033, doi.org/10.1038/s41591 -021-01336-3

16. Ben Sessa, "Why MDMA Therapy for Alcohol Use Disorder? And Why Now?" *Neuropharmacology* 142 (November 2018): 83–88, doi .org/10.1016/j.neuropharm.2017 .11.004

17. Ben Sessa et al., "First Study of Safety and Tolerability of 3,4-Methylenedioxy-methamphetamine-Assisted Psychotherapy in Patients With Alcohol Use Disorder," *Journal of Psychopharmacology* 35, no. 4 (April 2021): 375–383, doi.org/10 .1177/0269881121991792

THE DISSOCIATIVES

1. John Martin Corkery, "Ibogaine as a Treatment for Substance Misuse: Potential Benefits and Practical Dangers," *Progress in Brain Research* 242 (2018): 217–257, doi .org/10.1016/bs.pbr.2018.08.005, summarized at sciencedirect.com /topics/agricultural-and-biological -sciences/ibogaine

2. Samuel B. Obembe, "Ibogaine Therapy," section 6.5 in "Pharmacotherapy (Medication Therapy)," *Practical Skills and Clinical Management of Alcoholism and Drug Addiction* (2012): 79–95, doi.org/10.1016 /B978-0-12-398518-7.00006-7, summarized at sciencedirect.com /topics/agricultural-and -biological-sciences/ibogaine

3. Elaine Elisabetsky, "Ibogaine and Drug Addiction," section IX in "Traditional Medicines and the New Paradigm of Psychotropic Drug Action," *Advances in Phytomedicine* 1 (2002): 133–144, doi.org/10.1016/S1572-557X (02)80020-4, summarized at sciencedirect.com/topics /agricultural-and-biological -sciences/ibogaine

CHAPTER 6

1. Romaldas Mačiulaitis et al., "Ibogaine, an Anti-addictive Drug: Pharmacology and Time to Go Further in Development: A Narrative Review," *Human & Experimental Toxicology* 27, no. 3 (March 2008), 181–194, doi.org /10.1177/0960327107087802

2. *Encyclopedia Britannica*, "Bwiti, African Religion," accessed April 14, 2022, britannica.com/topic /Bwiti

3. Giorgio Samorini, "Adam, Eve and Iboga," *Integration* 4 (1993): 4–10, yumpu.com/en/document/read /25973702/adam-eve-and-iboga -giorgio-samorini-network

4. Vincent Ravalec, Mallendi, and Agnès Paicheler, *Iboga: The Visionary Root of African Shamanism* (Rochester, Vermont: Park Street, 2007), 14–15.

5. Ravalec, Mallendi, and Paicheler, *Iboga*, 15.

6. Ravalec, Mallendi, and Paicheler, *Iboga*, 16.

7. Emily J. Richer, "History of Ibogaine" in "Ibogaine and the Treatment of Opiate Addiction," *Complementary and Alternative Therapies and the Aging Population* (2009): 393–401, doi .org/10.1016/B978-0-12-374228 -5.00019-6, summarized at sciencedirect.com/topics /neuroscience/iboga

8. Ravalec, Mallendi, and Paicheler, *Iboga*, 115–116.

9. Ravalec, Mallendi, and Paicheler, *Iboga*, 24–27.

10. Ravalec, Mallendi, and Paicheler, *Iboga*, 24.

11. Ravalec, Mallendi, and Paicheler, *Iboga*, 118–119.

12. Ravalec, Mallendi, and Paicheler, *Iboga*, 119–120.

13. Kenneth R. Alper, Dana Beal, and Charles D. Kaplan, "A Contemporary History of Ibogaine in the United States and Europe," ch. 14 in *The Alkaloids: Chemistry and Biology* 56 (2001): 249–281, doi.org/10.1016/S0099-9598 (01)56018-6

14. Ravalec, Mallendi, and Paicheler, *Iboga*, 123–124.

15. "Howard Lotsof (RIP) Speaks About Ibogaine," *YouTube*, July 26, 2007, youtube.com/watch?v =TezytTw72Bg

16. Ravalec, Mallendi, and Paicheler, *Iboga*, 125.

17. Alper, Beal, and Kaplan, "Contemporary History."

18. Alper, Beal, and Kaplan, "Contemporary History."

19. Christine L. Mattson et al., "Trends and Geographic Patterns in Drug and Synthetic Opioid Overdose Deaths—United States, 2013–2019," *Morbidity and Mortality Weekly Report* 70, no. 6 (February 12, 2021): 202–207, doi .org/10.15585/mmwr.mm7006a4

20. Mathias Luz and Deborah C. Mash, "Evaluating the Toxicity and Therapeutic Potential of Ibogaine in the Treatment of Chronic Opioid Abuse," *Expert Opinion on Drug Metabolism & Toxicology* 17, no. 9 (2021): 1019–1022, doi.org/10 .1080/17425255.2021.1944099

21. U. Maas and S. Strubelt, "Fatalities After Taking Ibogaine in Addiction Treatment Could Be Related to Sudden Cardiac Death Caused by Autonomic Dysfunction," *Medical Hypotheses* 67, no. 4 (2006): 960–964, doi.org/10.1016/j.mehy.2006.02.050

22. Luz and Mash, "Evaluating the Toxicity and Therapeutic Potential."

23. Luz and Mash, "Evaluating the Toxicity and Therapeutic Potential."

24. Deborah C. Mash et al., "Ibogaine Detoxification Transitions Opioid and Cocaine Abusers Between Dependence and Abstinence: Clinical Observations and Treatment Outcomes," *Frontiers in Pharmacology* 9 (June 2018): article 529, doi.org/10.3389/fphar .2018.00529

25. Paul Glue et al., "Ascending-Dose Study of Noribogaine in Healthy Volunteers: Pharmacokinetics, Pharmacodynamics, Safety, and Tolerability," *Journal of Clinical Pharmacology* 55, no. 2 (February 2015): 189–194, doi.org/10.1002 /jcph.404

26. "Preliminary Efficacy and Safety of Ibogaine in the Treatment of Methadone Detoxification," *U.S. National Library of Medicine*, July 1, 2019, clinicaltrials.gov/ct2/show/NCT04003948

27. Kezia Parkins, "DemeRx and Atai Get MHRA Nod to Start Trial of Ibogaine for Opioid Use Disorder," *Clinical Trials Arena*, March 10, 2021, clinicaltrialsarena.com/news/ibogaine-demerx-atai-mhra-clinical-trial/

28. "A Study to Assess 18-Methoxycoronaridine (18-MC HCl) in Healthy Volunteers," *U.S. National Library of Medicine*, March 3, 2020, clinicaltrials.gov/ct2/show/NCT04292197

CHAPTER 7

1. Yan Yang et al., "Ketamine Blocks Bursting in the Lateral Habenula to Rapidly Relieve Depression," *Nature*, no. 554 (February 2018): 317–322, doi.org/10.1038/nature25509

2. Tao Yang et al., "The Role of BDNF on Neural Plasticity in Depression," *Frontiers in Cellular Neuroscience* 14 (April 2020): article 82, doi.org/10.3389/fncel.2020.00082

3. Linda Li and Phillip E. Vlisides, "Ketamine: 50 Years of Modulating the Mind," *Frontiers in Human Neuroscience* 10 (November 2016): article 612, doi.org/10.3389/fnhum.2016.00612

4. Edward F. Domino and David S. Warner, "Taming the Ketamine Tiger," *Anesthesiology* 113 (September 2010): 678–684, doi.org/10.1097/ALN.0b013e3181ed09a2

5. "KETAMINE HYDROCHLORIDE—Ketamine Hydrochloride Injection, Solution, Concentrate," Hospira Inc., revised March 2021, labeling.pfizer.com/ShowLabeling.aspx?id=4485

6. Georges Mion, "History of Anesthesia: The Ketamine Story—Past, Present, and Future," *European Journal of Anaesthesiology* 34, no. 9 (September 2017): 571–575, doi.org/10.1097/EJA.0000000000000638

7. P.F. White and M.R. Elig, "Intravenous Anesthetics," in Paul G. Barash et al., eds., *Clinical Anesthesia*, 6th ed. (Wolters Kluwer, 2013), 478–500.

8. "Committed to Breaking New Ground in the Understanding and Care of Psychiatric Conditions," *Clinical Trials at Yale*, website for the Yale School of Medicine, August 31, 2020, medicine.yale.edu/ycci/clinicaltrials/learnmore/ketamine/

9. Ewa Wajs et al., "Esketamine Nasal Spray Plus Oral Antidepressant in Patients With Treatment-Resistant Depression: Assessment of Long-Term Safety in a Phase 3, Open-Label Study (SUSTAIN-2)," *Journal of Clinical Psychiatry* 81, no. 3 (2020): article 19m12891, doi.org/10.4088/JCP.19m12891

10. Walter S. Marcantoni et al., "A Systematic Review and Meta-Analysis of the Efficacy of Intravenous Ketamine Infusion for Treatment Resistant Depression: January 2009–January 2019," *Journal of Affective Disorders* 277 (December 2020): 831–841, doi.org/10.1016/j.jad.2020.09.007

11. David A. Luckenbaugh et al., "Do the Dissociative Side Effects of Ketamine Mediate Its Anti-depressant Effects?," *Journal of Affective Disorders* 159 (April 2014): 56–61, doi.org/10.1016/j.jad.2014.02.017

12. Meryem Grabski et al., "Adjunctive Ketamine With Relapse Prevention–Based Psychological Therapy in the Treatment of Alcohol Use Disorder," *American Journal of Psychiatry* 179, no. 2 (February 2022): 152–162, doi.org/10.1176/appi.ajp.2021.21030277

13. Adele Lafrance and Reid Robison, "Psychedelics and Eating Disorders," *Eating Disorders Resource Catalogue*, January 23, 2021, edcatalogue.com/psychedelics-eating-disorders/

14. Terry Schwartz et al., "A Longitudinal Case Series of IM Ketamine for Patients With Severe and Enduring Eating Disorders and Comorbid Treatment-Resistant Depression," *Clinical Case Reports* 9, no. 5 (May 2021): article e03869, doi.org/10.1002/ccr3.3869

15. Paul Glue et al., "Safety and Efficacy of Maintenance Ketamine Treatment in Patients With Treatment-Refractory Generalised Anxiety and Social Anxiety Disorders," *Journal of Psychopharmacology* 32, no. 6 (2018): 663–667, doi.org/10.1177/0269881118762073

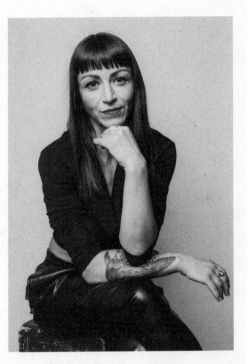

Author photo by Kristine Cofsky

Based on unceded Qayqayt territory in New Westminster, British Columbia, Amanda Siebert is an award-winning journalist and photographer and owes her life to the plants and fungi she writes about. She is also the author of *The Little Book of Cannabis: How Marijuana Can Improve Your Life.*